The Easiest Inst... Pressure Cookbook

must-have.

The New Way

to enjoy food with pressure cook

quick and easy 70+ delicious & healthy

recipes.

Vessava Venuda

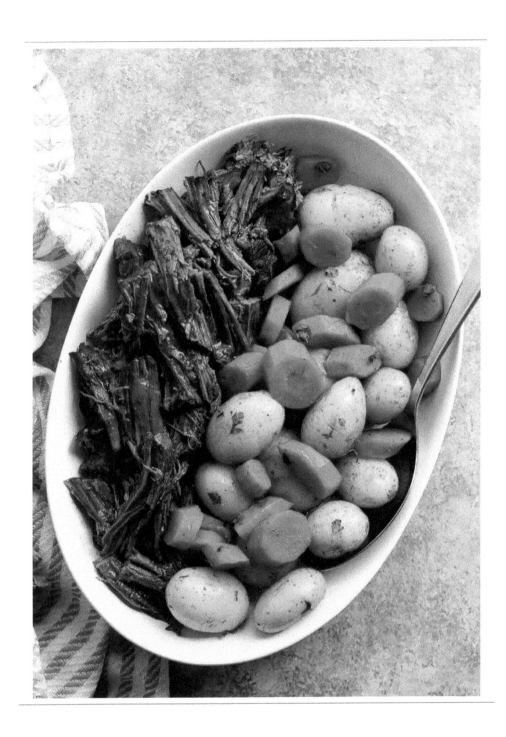

Table of Contents

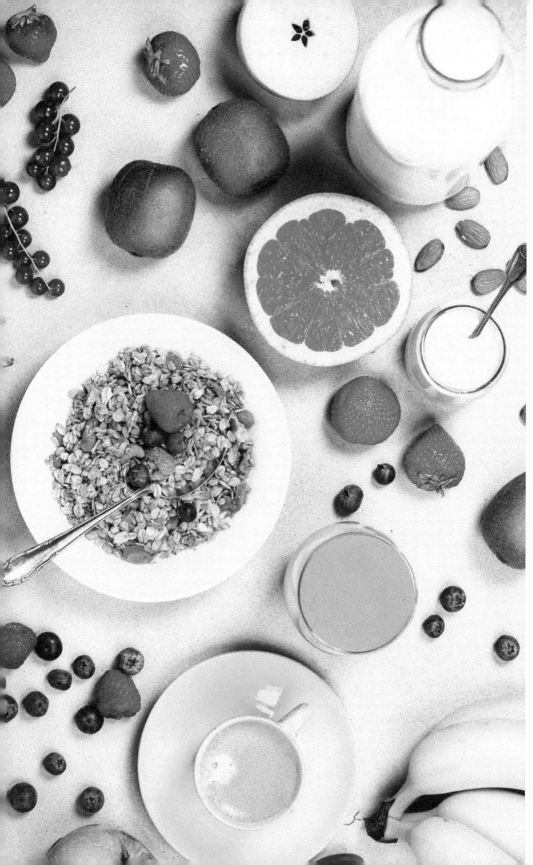

Breakfast Specials

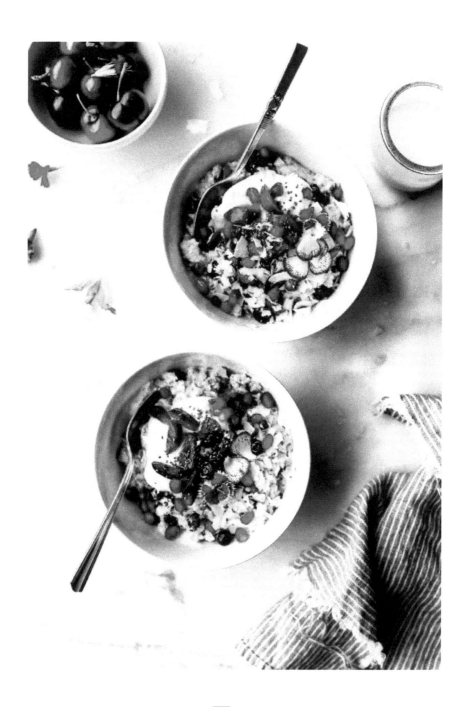

Egg & Bread Morning

Serving Yields: 4-6

Points Allotted - Smart Points: 4

Prep & Cooking Time: 18-20 minutes

Nutritional Macros Per Serving:

- **Calories**: 253
- **Protein Count**: 15 g
- **Fat Content**: 11.5 g
- **Carbs**: 22 g

List of Ingredients Needed:

- Large bread rolls (3)
- Grated cheddar cheese (7 oz.)
- Red chili flakes (.5 tsp.)
- Eggs (4)
- Sour cream (.5 tsp.)
- Butter (1 tbsp.)
- Salt (as desired)

Preparation Technique:

1. Slice the rolls into halves and remove part of the centers.

2. Whisk the salt, pepper, and sour cream in a mixing bowl. Mix in the eggs.

3. Lightly grease the Instant Pot and arrange the rolls in the pot, topping with the cheese and spice mixture (or other spices to your liking).

4. Lock-down the lid and seal the pressure valve. Select the steam function and adjust the timer for ten minutes.

5. When the time has elapsed, quick-release the pressure and serve.

Fajita Breakfast Casserole

Serving Yields: 2

Points Allotted - Smart Points: 2

Prep & Cooking Time: 12 minutes

Nutritional Macros Per Serving:

- **Calories**: 241

- **Protein Count**: 12 g

- **Fat Content**: 16 g

- **Carbs**: 11 g

List of Ingredients Needed:

- Onion (.5 cup)

- Bell peppers - sliced: Green, red, and orange (1.5 cups)

- Olive oil (1 tbsp.)

- Eggs (4)

Preparation Technique:

1. Use the sauté mode on the Instant Pot and pour in the oil. Wait for it to get hot.

2. Slice and toss in the garlic, bell peppers, and onions. Sauté the mixture for about five minutes until the edges of the onions and bell peppers start to caramelize, like fajitas.

3. Click the Instant Pot to the off position (to stop the sauté function) and transfer the peppers and onions to a round oven-safe pan that will fit inside. (Use a 2-quart soufflé pan, but any oven-safe dish would work.)

4. Gently crack four eggs and place them on top of the peppers so that the yolk is intact. Sprinkle it with salt and a portion of freshly cracked black pepper. Cover it with foil.

5. Make a sling using strips of heavy-duty foil, so the container can be easily removed from the hot pot.

6. Place a trivet in the Instant Pot insert and add one cup of water. Gently lower the covered dish to sit on top of the trivet. Lock the top into place to close.

7. Set the pot using the high-pressure function for two minutes. Quick-release the steam and pressure when it's done.

8. Remove the dish from the Instant Pot. Top with avocados, cilantro, and sliced limes as desired before serving.

Ham & Egg Frittata

Serving Yields: 4-6

Points Allotted - Smart Points: 2

Prep & Cooking Time: 18-20 minutes

Nutritional Macros Per Serving:

- **Calories**: 215

- **Protein Count**: 17.5 g

- **Fat Content**: 13 g

- **Carbs**: 6.5 g

List of Ingredients Needed:

- Olive oil (1 tsp.)

- Ham (8 oz.)

- Lemon zest (1 tbsp.)

- Salt (1 tsp)

- Parsley (.5 cup)

- Paprika (.5 tsp.)

- White pepper (1 tsp.)

- Eggs (7)

- Milk (.5 cup)

- Tomato (1)

Preparation Technique:

1. Chop the ham, tomato, and parsley. Set them aside for now.

2. Whisk the eggs with the paprika, salt, milk, pepper, and zest of lemon.

3. Toss into a mixer and add the ham and tomatoes.

4. Spritz the Instant Pot with oil and add the ham mixture, topped with parsley.

5. Securely close the top, sealing the valve.

6. Choose the steam mode, and set the timer for 10 minutes.

7. Once the time has elapsed, quick-release the built-up steam, open the lid carefully and serve.

Hard-Boiled Eggs

Serving Yields: 3

Points Allotted - Smart Points: 2 per egg

Prep & Cooking Time: 7 minutes

Nutritional Macros Per Serving:

- **Calories**: 126

- **Protein Count**: 11 g

- **Fat Content**: 8 g

- **Carbs**: 1 g

List of Ingredients Needed:

- Eggs (6)

- Water (1 cup)

Preparation Technique:

1. Place the metal rack inside the Instant Pot.

2. Places the eggs on the metal rack.

3. Pour one cup of water into the cooking pot.

4. Set the timer for five minutes.

5. Natural-release the built-up steam pressure for five minutes, then release the rest of the steam manually.

6. Place hard-boiled eggs in cold water.

7. When they are chilled, peel, and eat!

Healthy Starbucks 'Copycat' Red Pepper Egg Bites

Serving Yields: 7/14 bites/2 per serving

Points Allotted - Smart Points: 4

Prep & Cooking Time: 25 minutes

Nutritional Macros Per Serving:

- **Calories**: 259

- **Protein Count**: 20 g

- **Fat Content**: 16 g

- **Carbs**: 5 g

List of Ingredients Needed:

- Eggs (6)

- Cheddar cheese (.66 cup)

- Plain Greek yogurt 2% (.75 cup)

- Cottage cheese 2-4% (.75 cup)

- Red bell peppers (2 cups)

- Green onions (.33 cup)

- Turkey bacon (14 slices - cooked and chopped)

- Avocado/coconut/olive oil (1 tsp.)

Preparation Technique:

1. Pour a cup of water into the pot of the cooker and add the basket/trivet.

2. Grease the silicone molds with the oil so that the bites do not stick in the container.

3. Chop the onions and dice the peppers.

4. Fill each cup of the silicone mold halfway full of green onions, turkey bacon, and bell peppers.

5. In a blender, mix the egg, cheese, yogurt, and cottage cheese. Blend until it's smooth, about 30 seconds.

6. Pour the egg mixture in the silicone mold. Fill each cup to about ¼-inch below the brim. Cover it with foil.

7. Stack both trays on the trivet in the cooker. Rotate the top tray slightly to offset it so that the cups are not directly on top of each other.

8. Securely close the top and seal the pressure valve. Use the high-pressure mode - steam function - for about eight minutes. Natural-release the pressure.

9. Unplug the pot and remove the egg bites. Take off the foil and flip the mold upside down and cool it until the egg bites can be removed from the silicone tray without sticking.

10. Serve them warm and place any leftovers in the fridge for up to seven days. They can also be frozen for up to a month and reheated in the microwave for a minute.

Mini Frittata

Serving Yields: 3

Points Allotted - Smart Points: 3

Prep & Cooking Time: 12 minutes

Nutritional Macros Per Serving:

- **Calories**: 253

- **Protein Count**: 19.6 g

- **Fat Content**: 13.1 g

- **Carbs**: 13.9 g

List of Ingredients Needed:

- Turkey bacon (4 slices - chopped)

- Eggs (6)

- Salt and pepper (1 tsp. each)

- Small red potato (1)

- Bell pepper (half of 1)

- Small onion (half of 1)

- Milk (.25 cup)

- Cheddar cheese (.25 cup)

- Ceramic ramekins (3)

Preparation Technique:

1. Pour one cup of water into the cooker and add the basket/trivet.

2. Cover the ramekins with a piece of aluminum foil to place them on the trivet.

3. Set the timer for ten minutes using the high-pressure function. Be careful and quick-release the built-up steam. Wait for a few minutes before serving them.

4. Place any leftovers into a plastic zipper-type bag to enjoy later in the week. Storage in the fridge is recommended. Reheat for 60 seconds in the microwave.

Peaches & "Dream" Oatmeal

Serving Yields: 4

Points Allotted - Smart Points:

Green: 6/Blue: 5/ Purple: 1

Prep & Cooking Time: 50 minutes

Nutritional Macros Per Serving:

- **Calories**: 245
- **Protein Count**: 8 g
- **Fat Content**: 5.5 g
- **Carbs**: 40 g

List of Ingredients Needed:

- Unsweetened vanilla almond milk (2 cups)
- Chopped peaches (fresh/ frozen and thawed (2 cups)
- Vanilla extract (1 tbsp.)
- Chia seeds (1.5 tbsp.)
- Steel-cut oats (1 cup)
- Cinnamon (2 tsp.)
- No-calorie sweetener (5 packets)
- Salt (.25 tsp.)

Preparation Technique:

1. Gently spritz the Instant Pot (IP) with cooking oil spray.

2. Mix in each of the fixings, and stir well.

3. Securely lock-down the top. Using the *manual* mode, and set the timer for 13 minutes.

4. Cook until the timer buzzes and do a natural release of the pressure for 10 minutes. Gently stir the oats before serving.

Power-Packed Buckwheat Porridge with Creamed Spinach

Serving Yields: 4

Points Allotted - Smart Points: 2

Prep & Cooking Time: 15 minutes

Nutritional Macros Per Serving:

- **Calories**: 184

- **Protein Count**: 2 g

- **Fat Content**: 6 g

- **Carbs**: 25 g

List of Ingredients Needed:

- Sliced banana (1 cup)

- Raw buckwheat groats (1 cup)

- Water (2 cups)

- Rice milk (1 cup)

- Raisins (.5 cup)

- Cinnamon powder (1 tsp.)

- Vanilla (.5 tsp.)

- Optional: Nuts of choice for topping (add the calories)

Preparation Technique:

1. Rinse the buckwheat and dump it into the Instant Pot.

2. Slice and mix in the banana, raisins, vanilla, cinnamon, water, and milk.

3. Set the Instant Pot at high pressure for ten minutes.

4. Natural-release the steam pressure and open the top. Pour in additional milk if desired. Stir and serve with optional nuts as desired.

Lunch Favourites

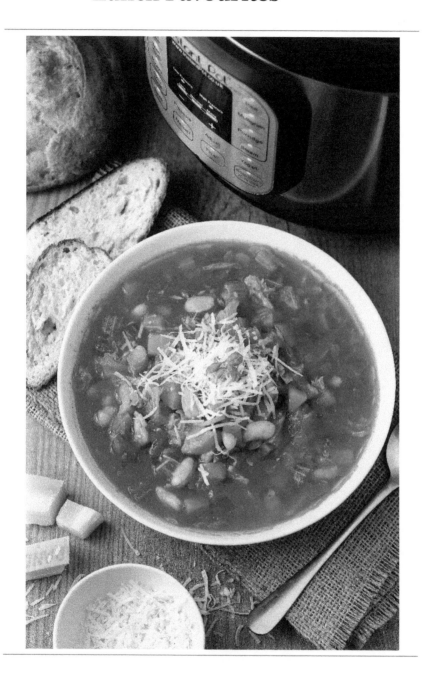

Lentil Soup With Sweet Potato

Serving Yields: 4

Points Allotted - Smart Points: 4

Prep & Cooking Time: 47 minutes

Nutritional Macros Per Serving:

- **Calories**: 187.8

- **Protein Count**: 9 g

- **Fat Content**: 2.6 g

- **Carbs**: 41 g

List of Ingredients Needed:

- Olive oil (2 tsp.)

- Garlic cloves (4)

- Yellow onion (half of 1)

- Celery (1 large stalk)

- Paprika (1 tsp.)

- Ground cumin (1 tsp.)

- Red pepper flakes (.5 tsp.)

- Green lentils (1 cup)

- Salt (.5 tsp.)

- Sweet potatoes - .5-inch diced (.75 lb.)

- Low-sodium vegetable broth (3.5 cups)

- Water (1 cup)

- Petite diced tomatoes (14 oz. can)

- Spinach leaves (4 oz./4 cups packed)

- Freshly cracked black pepper and salt (as desired)

Preparation Technique:

1. Use the sauté function to warm the oil for about 30 seconds.

2. Chop the onion and celery and toss into the Instant P

3. Sauté for about four minutes. Mince, and add the garlic, paprika, cumin, pepper flakes, and black pepper.

4. Dice and stir in the potatoes, lentils, water, broth, and diced tomatoes.

5. Stir it thoroughly and lock-down the top. Use the high-pressure function to cook for 12 minutes.

6. Natural-release the built-up pressure for ten minutes, and quick-release the rest of the steam at that point.

7. Stir in the spinach until it's wilted and sprinkle with the seasonings to your liking before serving.

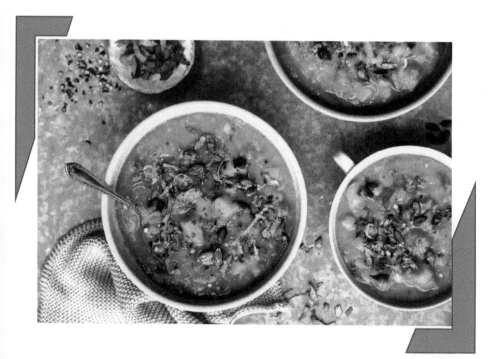

Mexican Lentil Soup

Serving Yields: 6

Points Allotted - Smart Points: 0

Prep & Cooking Time: 20 minutes

Nutritional Macros Per Serving:

- **Calories**: 270

- **Protein Count**: 15 g

- **Fat Content**: 3 g

- **Carbs**: 46 g

List of Ingredients Needed:

- Olive oil (1 tbsp.)

- Onion (2)

- Peppers (2)

- Carrots (3)

- Optional: Bay leaf

- Garlic puree (1 tsp.)

- Cumin (1.5 tsp.)

- Smoked paprika (1.5 tsp.)

- Chili powder (1 pinch or to taste)

- Green lentils (1.5 cups)

- Vegetable stock (3 cups)

- Finely chopped tomatoes (2 - 14 oz. cans)

- Salt as desired

- Chopped Coriander/cilantro (6 tbsp.)

Preparation Technique:

1. Peel and finely chop the tomatoes, peppers, onions, and carrots. Pick and rinse the lentils.

2. Select the Instant Pot sauté setting, and add the oil to heat. Toss in the bay leaf, onions, carrots, and peppers. Sauté for four to five minutes. Turn off the pot and mix in the chili, cumin, paprika, and garlic.

3. Stir well and add the veggie stock, lentils, salt, and tomatoes.

4. Securely lock-down the top and prepare for seven minutes. Once the timer buzzes, wait 15 minutes for a natural-release of pressure. Then, quick-release the rest of the built-up steam. Stir in the coriander and serve.

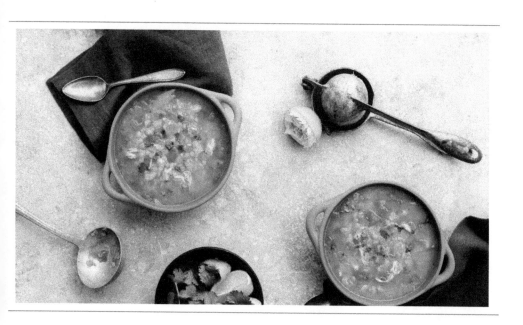

Mushroom Soup – Vegan Style

Serving Yields: 4

Points Allotted - Smart Points: 3

Prep & Cooking Time: 40 minutes

Nutritional Macros Per Serving:

- **Calories**: 108

- **Protein Count**: 4.8 g

- **Fat Content**: 2.4 g

- **Carbs**: 12.7 g

List of Ingredients Needed:

- Olive oil (12 tsp.)

- Onion (1 medium)

- Celery (1 large stalk)

- Carrot (1 large)

- Garlic (4 cloves)

- Shiitake & Cremini mushrooms (8 oz. each)

- Dried thyme (1 tsp)

- Black pepper (.5 tsp.)

- Vegetable broth (3 cups)

- Coconut milk (.66 cup)

- Kosher salt (.5 tsp.)

Preparation Technique:

1. Chop the carrots, celery, and garlic. Slice the mushrooms.

2. Prepare the Instant Pot using the sauté function, adding the oil to heat.

3. Chop the carrots, onions, and celery. Toss them into the Instant Pot and sauté them for about three to four minutes. Toss in the garlic, thyme, pepper, and both types of mushrooms. Sauté for about two to three minutes. Stir in the salt and broth.

4. Securely close the top. Set the timer to ten minutes using the high setting. When it beeps, quick-release the steam.

5. Dump the soup and milk into a blender, mixing until almost smooth.

6. Pour it into a bowl and repeat with the second half of the soup. Reheat the soup in the Instant Pot as needed using the sauté function.

Split Pea & Ham Soup

Serving Yields: 8

Points Allotted - Smart Points:

Green: 8/Blue: 1/ Purple: 1

Prep & Cooking Time: 25 minutes

Nutritional Macros Per Serving:

- **Calories**: 182

- **Protein Count**: 17 g

- **Fat Content**: 1.5 g

- **Carbs**: 39 g

List of Ingredients Needed:

- Dry green split peas (1 lb.)

- Carrots (2 large)

- Onion (1 medium)

- Celery (.25 cup)

- Cloves of garlic (2)

- Olive oil (1 tsp.)

- Leftover ham bone

- Water (6 cups)

- Better Than Bouillon /1 cube (1 tbsp.)

- Bay leaf (1)

- Leftover ham (4 oz.)

- For the Garnish: Chopped chives

Preparation Technique:

1. Rinse the peas thoroughly using chilled water. Peel and dice the carrots, onions, celery, and garlic.

2. Warm the Instant Pot and oil using the sauté function.

3. Toss in the onions, carrots, celery, and garlic and sauté for four to five minutes.

4. Add the water, peas, ham bone, bay leaf, and chicken bouillon. Put the top on the cooker and set the Instant Pot using the high-pressure setting (15 min.).

5. Natural-release the built-up steam pressure (10 min.) and open the top. Discard the bone and bay leaf. Stir and wait a few minutes as the soup will thicken while you wait.

6. Meanwhile, dice and sauté the ham using a hot skillet to make it crunchy if desired. Use it as a tasty topping on the soup with a dash of chives.

Steak Soup

Serving Yields: 8

Points Allotted - Smart Points: 3

Prep & Cooking Time: 25 minutes

Nutritional Macros Per Serving:

- **Calories**: 364

- **Protein Count**: 30 g

- **Fat Content**: 7 g

- **Carbs**: 24 g

List of Ingredients Needed:

- Steak, or stew meat (1 lb.)

- Onion (1)

- Carrots (2)

- Celery (2 stalks)

- Sweet peppers (4 diced) or (1 large bell pepper)

- Mushrooms - cremini/button (8 oz.)

- Garlic powder (2 tbsp.)

- Thyme (1 tsp.)

- Celtic sea salt (2 tsp.)

- Bay leaf (1)

- Oregano (2 tsp.)

- Crushed tomatoes (1 cup)

- Water (2 cups)

- Beef stock (2 cups)

Preparation Technique:

1. Set the Instant Pot to the sauté function.

2. Discard the fat from the stew meat and brown it in the cooker.

3. Dice and add the onion, celery, peppers, carrots, and cook until softened.

4. Thinly slice and add the mushrooms, cook until soft.

5. Add the spices, salt, water, and stock and cover the Instant Pot, setting to seal.

6. Cook on soup setting for 15 minutes. Release the built-up steam and serve hot.

Stuffed Pepper Soup

Serving Yields: 8

Points Allotted - Smart Points: 2

Prep & Cooking Time: 18-23 minutes

Nutritional Macros Per Serving:

- **Calories**: 130

- **Protein Count**: 16 g

- **Fat Content**: 2 g

- **Carbs**: 14 g

List of Ingredients Needed:

- Extra-lean ground turkey/beef (1 lb.)

- Onion (1 cup)

- Diced tomatoes with roasted garlic and onions (14.5 oz.)

- Tomato sauce (15 oz.)

- Bell peppers - green and red (3 cups)

- Broth - Low sodium/Water (2 cups)

- Brown rice (.5 cup - dry and rinsed)

- Garlic (1 clove)

- Oregano (2 tsp.)

- Black pepper (.25 tsp.)

Preparation Technique:

1. Spray the Instant Pot with oil and sauté the ground turkey.

2. Chop the onion, peppers, and add all of the fixings into the Instant Pot. Tightly lock-down the top. Use the high-pressure setting and set the timer for 8 minutes.

3. Quick-release the built-up pressure when it's done.

Taco Soup

Serving Yields: 6

Points Allotted - Smart Points:

Green: 6/Blue: 0/ Purple: 0

Prep & Cooking Time: 20 minutes

Nutritional Macros Per Serving:

- **Calories**: 306

- **Protein Count**: 28 g

- **Fat Content**: 3 g

- **Carbs**: 44 g

List of Ingredients Needed:

- Chicken breast (1 lb.)

- Onion (1)

- Pinto beans (14.5 oz. can

- Black beans (14.5 oz. can)

- Garlic cloves (2)

- Corn (14.5 oz. can)

- Canned diced tomatoes with green chilies - not drained (14.5 oz.)

- Chicken broth - Fat-free (2 cups)

- Taco seasoning (1.25 oz.)

Preparation Technique:

1. Remove the bones and skin from the chicken. Mince the garlic and onion. Drain the corn and beans.

2. Use the soup setting (8 min.) and then natural-release the pressure to serve.

Turkey Pumpkin Chili

Serving Yields:

Points Allotted - Smart Points:

Green: 6/Blue: 4/ Purple: 4

Prep & Cooking Time: 45 minutes

Nutritional Macros Per Serving:

- **Calories**: 300
- **Protein Count**: 27 g
- **Fat Content**: 8 g
- **Carbs**: 31 g

List of Ingredients Needed:

- Yellow onion (1 large - about 2 cups)
- Bell pepper, yellow, red, or orange (1 medium)
- Garlic (6 cloves or 0.75 tsp. garlic powder)
- 90-93 % lean ground turkey/chicken (1.33 lb.)
- Canned diced tomatoes with liquid (28 oz.)
- Canned white beans (15 oz.)
- Tomato paste -no salt added (.25 cup)
- Pumpkin puree (14-oz. can)
- Vegetable/chicken broth - Reduced-sodium (1 cup)
- Cumin (2.5 tsp.)
- Cocoa powder (1 tbsp.)
- Chili powder (2 tbsp.)
- Ground cinnamon (1.5 tsp.) or Pumpkin pie spice (1 tbsp.)
- Kosher salt (1 tsp.)
- Optional: Cayenne pepper (.5 tsp.)

- Freshly cracked black pepper (.5 tsp.)

- Baby spinach leaves (4 cups)

Optional:

- Avocado

- Sour cream or Nonfat plain Greek yogurt

- Cilantro

Preparation Technique:

1. Liberally coat the Instant Pot using a cooking oil spray. Press the sauté function on the Instant Pot.

2. Rinse and drain the beans. Set them aside in a colander.

3. Dice and mix in the onion and bell pepper to the cooker. Sauté, occasionally stirring, until the onion softens (7 min.).

4. Add in the garlic, stir everything together, and cook until fragrant (30 seconds).

5. Add the ground turkey or chicken and sauté it for about six to seven minutes.

6. Pour in the diced tomatoes, pumpkin puree, tomato paste, beans, broth, chili powder, cinnamon/pumpkin pie spice, cocoa powder, cumin, black pepper, and cayenne pepper. Stir thoroughly.

7. Prepare using the high setting for 15 minutes. When it's done, natural-release the steam pressure for 10 minutes and add the spinach. Stir it thoroughly before serving.

Vegetable Noodle Soup

Serving Yields: 4

Points Allotted - Smart Points: 4

Prep & Cooking Time: 18 minutes

Nutritional Macros Per Serving:

- **Calories**: 171
- **Protein Count**: 5 g
- **Fat Content**: 0.7 g
- **Carbs**: 34.1 g

List of Ingredients Needed:

- Onion (1)
- Large carrot (1)
- Small sweet potato (half of 1)
- Garlic (1 clove)
- Frozen sweet corn (.5 cup)
- Tomato paste (1 tbsp.)
- Garlic powder (.25 tsp.)
- Paprika (1 tsp.)
- Chili powder (.25 tsp.)
- Dried basil, oregano, thyme and parsley (1 pinch of each)
- Salt and black pepper (as desired)
- Vegetable or chicken stock (5 cups/1.2 liters)
- Uncooked pasta of choice (3.5 oz. 100 g)
- Spinach (4 handfuls)

Preparation Technique:

1. Warm the Instant Pot using the sauté function. Lightly spritz with a cooking oil spray.

2. Finely chop the onion, potato, and carrot. Mince/crush the garlic clove.

3. Toss in the onions, garlic, and carrots to sauté for two minutes to soften.

4. Mix in the sweet potato, tomato paste, and spices, stirring well to coat.

5. Pour in the stock, corn, and pasta. Securely lock the lid and prepare the soup for four minutes using the high-pressure setting.

6. When the timer buzzes, quick-release the built-up steam pressure.

7. Open the top of the Instant Pot, and fold in the spinach, black pepper, and salt.

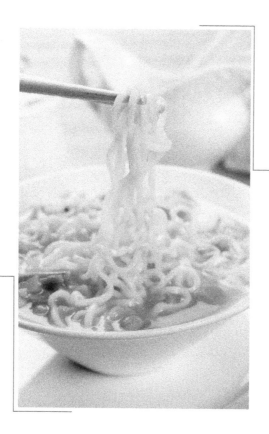

Vegetarian Chili

Serving Yields: 8

Points Allotted - Smart Points: 2

Prep & Cooking Time: 30 minutes

Nutritional Macros Per Serving:

- **Calories**: 34
- **Protein Count**: 1 g
- **Fat Content**: 0 g
- **Carbs**: 7 g

List of Ingredients Needed:

- Black beans (15 oz. can)
- Kidney beans (15.5 oz. can)
- Pinto beans (16 oz. can)
- Diced tomatoes (20 oz. can)
- Onion (1)
- Yellow, green & orange bell pepper (half of each)
- Water (5 cups)
- Vegetable bouillon cubes (2)
- Black pepper (.5 tsp.)
- Chili powder (2 tbsp.)
- Cayenne pepper (.5 tsp.)
- Garlic powder (2 tsp.)
- Dried oregano (1 tsp.)
- Onion powder (2 tsp.)
- Salt (1 tsp. or as desired)

Preparation Technique:

1. Warm the Instant Pot using the sauté function add in oil. Dice and add in the onions and bell peppers. Cook it for

about five minutes or
until they are tender.

2. Add in the pinto beans, black beans, diced tomatoes,
   kidney beans, seasonings, and water. Stir well to
   combine.

3. Securely close the top and set for 15 minutes using the
   high-pressure setting. Natural-release the pressure when
   it's done (10 min.).

4. Serve with optional toppings of lime wedges, diced green
   onion, cilantro, avocado, sour cream, or cheese.

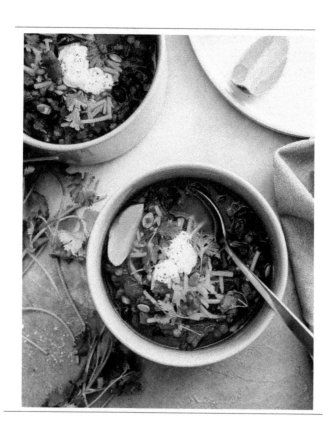

Vietnamese Chicken Soup

Serving Yields: 2-3

Points Allotted - Smart Points: 8

Prep & Cooking Time: 48-50 minutes

Nutritional Macros Per Serving:

- **Calories**: 380

- **Protein Count**: 45 g

- **Fat Content**: 3.5 g

- **Carbs**: 40 g

List of Ingredients Needed:

- Onion (1 small in quarters)

- Toasted coriander seeds (.5 tbsp.)

- Chicken pieces - skin-on - bone-in (1 lb.)

- Grated ginger (1 small chunk)

- Cardamom pods (.5 tsp.)

- Chopped lemongrass stalk (half 1)

- Cinnamon stick (half of 1)

- Cloves (2)

- Fish sauce (2 tbsp.)

- Chopped bok choy (half of 1)

- Spiralized Daikon root (half of 1

- Chopped green onions (1 tbsp.)

Preparation Technique:

1. Just pop the ingredients in the Instant Pot. Stir and loc the top in place.

2. Prepare the soup for 30 minutes. Once it's done, qu release the steam pressure slowly open the top.

3. Shred the chicken and add back into the cooker for everything to reheat. Stir a serve it with a garnish of chopped onions.

White Bean & Bacon Soup

Serving Yields: 6

Points Allotted - Smart Points: 5

Green: 5/Blue: 1

Prep & Cooking Time: 55 minutes

Nutritional Macros Per Serving:

- **Calories**: 225
- **Protein Count**: 16 g
- **Fat Content**: 2 g
- **Carbs**: 40 g

List of Ingredients Needed:

- White beans (3 - 15 oz. cans)
- Bacon (6 slices)
- Onions (1.5 cups)
- Carrots (.75 cups)
- Celery (.5 cup)
- Tomato paste (2 tbsp.)
- Reduced-sodium chicken broth - ex. 32 oz. carton of Swanson's (4 cups)
- Italian seasonings (1 tsp.) or Oregano and basil (0.5 tsp. each)
- Red pepper flakes (.125 tsp.)
- Black pepper (as desired)
- Optional for the Garnish: Chives or scallions - chopped

Preparation Technique:

1. Rinse and drain the beans and add them with one cup of water into a blender.

2. Warm the Instant Pot using the sauté function and add the bacon to cook until it's crispy. Stir often. Set aside on paper towels and blot.

3. Chop and add in the celery, carrots, and onions to the pot and sauté until softened (5 min.).

4. Mix in the pureed beans, tomato paste, broth, Italian seasonings, red pepper flakes, and black pepper.

5. Secure the lid on the Instant Pot and cook the soup for 20 minutes using the high-pressure setting. Natural-release the steam pressure (10-15 min.).

6. Pour 2.5 cups of soup into the blender. Puree it until its thickened and mix it back into the pot of soup.

7. To Serve: Ladle 1.5 cups into each bowl and top with a portion of crumbled bacon. Top with chives, as desired.

White Chili Chicken

Serving Yields: 4 - 2 cups per serving

Points Allotted - Smart Points: 2

Prep & Cooking Time: 55 minutes

Nutritional Macros Per Serving:

- **Calories**: 607

- **Protein Count**: 96 g

- **Fat Content**: 13 g

- **Carbs**: 23 g

List of Ingredients Needed:

- Frozen chicken breast (2 large or 1.5 - 2 lb.)

- White beans (1 cup dried - washed but not soaked)

- Green Chilis chopped I used poblano (3 fresh /about 1 cup)

- Jalapenos (2 chopped)

- Red bell pepper chopped (1 large or about 1 cup)

- Yellow onion (1 chopped about .5 cup)

- Minced garlic (4 cloves)

- Cumin (.5 tbsp.)

- Chili powder (.5 tbsp.)

- Pepper (.5 tsp.)

- Chicken stock (2 cups)

- Almond milk - unsweetened (1 cup)

- Greek yogurt - unflavored (.75 cup)

Preparation Technique:

1.   Dump everything into the Instant Pot except the yogurt and frozen chicken.

2.   Stir to mix up the seasoning.

3.   Place the frozen chicken on top so that you can easily shred it when it is done cooking.

4.   Securely close the lid. Prepare the chili for 45 minutes using the bean function (high-pressure setting). Natural-release the pressure for at least 10 minutes before doing a quick-release.

5.   Scoop the chicken out of the cooker and place it onto a chopping block, shred it, and add it back to the chili.

6.   Switch the Instant Pot to sauté function. Mix in the yogurt. Simmer for another 10-15 minutes to allow the chili to thicken if desired.

7.   Top with cheese, cilantro, and avocado to serve.

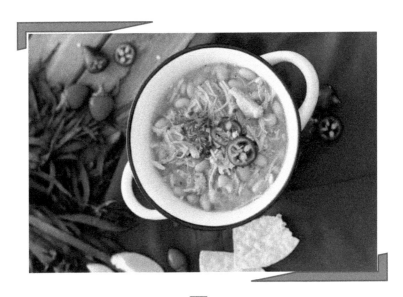

Zero Point Bean Soup

Serving Yields: 10

Points Allotted - Smart Points: 0

Prep & Cooking Time: 1.5 hours

Nutritional Macros Per Serving:

- **Calories**: 259

- **Protein Count**: 19 g

- **Fat Content**: 1 g

- **Carbs**: 39 g

List of Ingredients Needed:

- Olive oil (1 tsp.)

- Onion (1 medium)

- Celery (2 stalks)

- Cloves of garlic (3)

- Hurst's 15 Bean Soup Blend (20 oz. bag)

- Water (4 cups)

- Chicken broth - Low-sodium (4 cups)

- Red bell pepper (1)

- Large carrots (4)

- Worcestershire (2 tbsp.)

- Chili powder (2 tsp.)

- Bay leaves (2)

- Dried parsley (1 tbsp.)

- Dijon mustard (2 tbsp.)

- Optional: Liquid smoke (1 tsp.)

- Diced tomatoes with liquid (14.5 oz. can)

- Lemon juice (3 tbsp.)

- Salt and pepper (to your liking)

- Suggested: 6-quart Instant Pot

Preparation Technique:

1. Remove the seasonings from the beans and rinse them thoroughly.

2. Use the sauté mode on the Instant Pot to warm it and pour in the oil. Chop and add the onion, celery, and garlic.

3. Sauté them for four to five minutes, stirring often.

4. Add each of the fixings, excluding the tomatoes, lemon juice, salt, and pepper.

5. Securely lock the top and cook for 45 minutes using the high-pressure setting.

6. Once the cooking cycle is complete, natural-release the pressure for 20 minutes, then quick-release any remaining pressure.

7. Pour in the canned tomatoes and lemon juice, salt, and pepper as desired.

8. Mash some of the beans to thicken the soup if desired.

Poultry

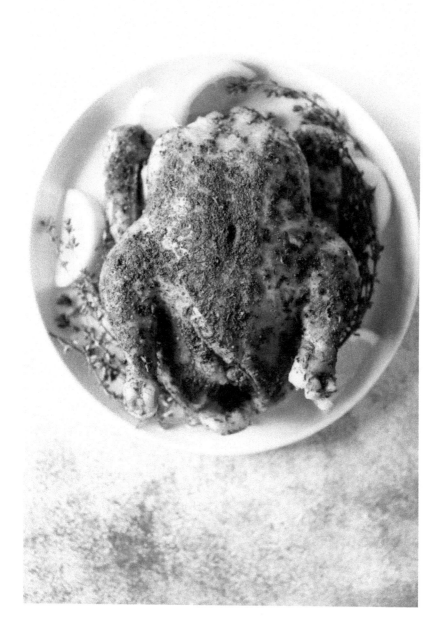

Garlic & Herb Chicken

Serving Yields: 6/0.75 cup each

Points Allotted - Smart Points:

Green: 2/Blue: 3 Purple: 0/Old Plan 3

Prep & Cooking Time: 35 minutes

Nutritional Macros Per Serving:

- **Calories**: 143

- **Protein Count**: 26 g

- **Fat Content**: 3 g

- **Carbs**: 1 g

List of Ingredients Needed:

- Raw boneless skinless chicken breast (1.5 lb.)

- Dried oregano (.5 tsp.)

- Onion powder (1 tsp.)

- Dried parsley (.5 tsp.)

- Dried basil (.5 tsp.)

- Black pepper & salt (.25 tsp. each)

- Garlic powder (1 tsp.)

- Chicken broth (2 cups)

Preparation Technique:

1. Arrange the chicken in the Instant Pot. Pour in the chicken broth and seasonings.

2. Securely close the lid, sealing the valve, and set the timer for eight minutes.

3. Quick-release the steam pressure and place the chicken into a large bowl, draining the broth. Shred the prepared chicken using two forks or your hands, and serve

Goulash

Serving Yields: 6

Points Allotted - Smart Points:

Prep & Cooking Time: 15 minutes

Nutritional Macros Per Serving:

- **Calories**: 190

- **Protein Count**: 22 g

- **Fat Content**: 2 g

- **Carbs**: 23 g

List of Ingredients Needed:

- Ground turkey (1 lb.)

- Zucchini (1 cup - chopped)

- Pasta whole wheat (1 cup)

- Bell peppers - chopped (1 cup)

Only include seasonings if you're using canned tomatoes:

- Minced garlic (1 tbsp.)

- Italian seasoning (2.5 tbsp.)

- Minced onions (1 tbsp.)

- Bay leaves (2)

- Jarred sauce OR Crushed tomatoes (14 oz.)

- Water (14 oz. - you'll be filling the tomato can with water)

  Optional: (If used, omit seasonings and tomatoes)

- Pasta sauce - no added sugar (1 jar)

Preparation Technique:

1. Program the Instant Pot setting to sauté and cook the ground turkey until it's done.

2. Note: If you're using jarred pasta sauce, skip the seasonings. Add garlic, minced onions, Italian seasoning, and two bay leaves. Toss in chopped zucchini and bell peppers.

3. Mix so that the seasonings and veggies are distributed.

4. Pour 8 ounces of dry pasta, can of crushed tomatoes (or a jar of pasta sauce), and fill the can back up with water and pour that over the veggies.

5. Stir until the pasta is thoroughly mixed with the sauce. Secure the lid and set the cooker using high pressure for three minutes. Use the quick-release method to release the pressure.

6. Stir it and let the goulash cool for a few minutes.

7. Top with cheese if desired and serve.

Honey Dijon Chicken

Serving Yields: 2

Points Allotted - Smart Points: 3

Prep & Cooking Time: 60 minutes

Nutritional Macros Per Serving:

- **Calories**: 786

- **Protein Count**: 98 g

- **Fat Content**: 34 g

- **Carbs**: 14 g

List of Ingredients Needed:

- Olive oil (3 tbsp.)

- Chicken breast (2 lb.)

- Dried thyme (1 tsp.)

- Small white onion (half of 1 - .25 cup)

- Garlic (2 cloves)

- Chicken broth (.5 cup)

- Honey (1 tbsp.)

- White wine or more chicken broth (.25 cup)

- Dijon mustard (2 tbsp.)

- Salt and pepper (to your liking)

Preparation Technique:

1. Set the Instant Pot to heat using the sauté mode for 10 minutes.

2. Use a mallet to flatten the chicken into a one-inch thickness. Season both sides using the thyme and salt.

Optional Step: Marinate the chicken in broth and wine for at least 20 minutes or up to 24 hours in the refrigerator.

3. Pour two tablespoons of oil into the cooker to heat using the sauté mode.

4. Add the chicken and sauté each side until browned (one minute

per side). Remove the
chicken and set it aside
for now.

5. Pour the remainder of the oil into the pot. Chop and
   add the onion. Sauté, often stirring, until the onion
   is translucent (3-5 min.).

6. Mince and add the garlic. Stir the mixture for
   another 30 seconds.

7. Arrange the chicken in the Instant Pot with the
   wine, mustard, and broth.

8. Secure the lid and set the timer for five minutes on
   the manual setting, and quick-release the steam
   when it's done.

9. Carefully remove the lid and set aside the chicken
   breast.

10. Program the Instant Pot to sauté and add honey to
    the remaining liquid to create a sauce. Stir
    frequently until the gravy-like consistency is
    reached.

11. Pour sauce over
    the chicken and
    serve.

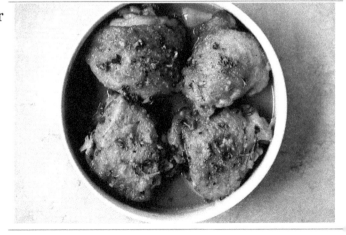

Honey Garlic Chicken

Serving Yields: 6

Points Allotted - Smart Points:

Green: 6/Blue: 6/ Purple: 6

Prep & Cooking Time: 30 minutes

Nutritional Macros Per Serving:

- **Calories**: 234

- **Protein Count**: 30 g

- **Fat Content**: 6 g

- **Carbs**: 13 g

List of Ingredients Needed:

- Chicken thighs (2 lb.)

- Low-sodium soy sauce (.33 cup)

- Ketchup - no-sugar-added (.25 cup)

- Honey (3 tbsp.)

- Garlic cloves (4)

Preparation Technique:

1. Remove the bones and skin from the chicken, and toss them into the bottom of the Instant Pot. Mince the garlic and toss it in with the rest of the fixings to create the sauce.

2. Pour the sauce over the chicken and stir. Securely lock the top and program the timer for 20 minutes using the high setting. Once it is finished cooking, quick-release the steam pressure.

3. Shred the chicken using two forks. If needed, you can thicken the sauce using a touch of cornstarch. It will depend on the liquid content of the thighs as to how much of it will be needed.

Indian Chicken Vindaloo

Serving Yields: 4

Points Allotted - Smart Points: 6

Prep & Cooking Time: 30 minutes

Nutritional Macros Per Serving:

- **Calories**: 199

- **Protein Count**: 23 g

- **Fat Content**: 8 g

- **Carbs**: 7 g

List of Ingredients Needed:

- Diced onion (1 cup)

- Garlic cloves (5)

- Minced ginger (2-3 slices)

- Oil (1 tbsp.)

- White vinegar (.25 cup)

- Chopped tomato (1 cup)

- Salt (1 tsp.)

- Garam masala (1 tsp.)

- Smoked paprika (1 tsp.)

- Cayenne pepper (.5 to 2 tsp.)

- Ground cumin (.5 tsp.)

- Ground coriander (.5 tsp.)

- Turmeric (.5 tsp.

- Water (.25 cup)

- Boneless- skinless chicken thighs (1 lb.)

Preparation Technique:

1. Mince/dice the ginger garlic, and onions and toss them into a microwave-safe bowl. Add the oil to the Instant Pot and set it to sauté.

2. Add the veggies to the hot cooker and sauté for 5-7 minutes.

3. Add it to a blender with the rest of the fixings except for the chicken, turmeric, and water. Mix into a smooth goo.

4. Coat the chicken with the blend. Rinse the blender with the water (¼ cup) and add it to the chicken.

5. Now, add the turmeric to marinate for at least half of an hour or up to eight hours.

6. Once you are ready to prepare it, dump all of the fixings into the Instant Pot for five minutes using the high-pressure setting.

7. Natural-release the built-up steam pressure for ten minutes, then, quick-release the rest.

8. Cook the sauce longer or use it as it is - before serving.

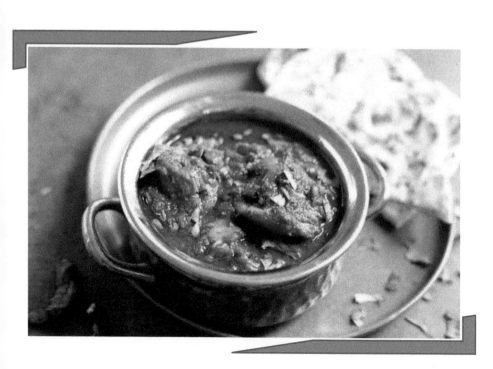

Low-Fat Chicken Wings – Instant Pot - Oven

- Butt Rub BBQ Seasoning/any dry barbecue seasoning blend

Serving Yields: 8

Points Allotted - Smart Points: 2

Prep & Cooking Time: 30 minutes

Nutritional Macros Per Serving:

- **Calories**: 63

- **Protein Count**: 5.5 g

- **Fat Content**: 4.4 g

- **Carbs**: 0 g

List of Ingredients Needed:

- Chicken drumettes (3 lb.)

- Franks Red Hot Sauce (2 tbsp.)

- Water (1 cup)

Preparation Technique:

1. Add one cup of water into the Instant Pot and add the trivet rack. Lightly spritz a tray with a portion of cooking oil.

2. Toss the wings into a container with one teaspoon of seasoning and the hot sauce. Toss well and place them on the top of the rack.

3. Securely close the top and set the timer for ten minutes (high-pressure setting).

4. When it's done, quick-release the pressure and remove the wings. Sprinkle them with seasoning and place on a baking pan. Broil for five to eight minutes until they're crispy as you like them.

Orange Chicken

Serving Yields: 4

Points Allotted - Smart Points: 9

Prep & Cooking Time: 27 minutes

Nutritional Macros Per Serving:

- **Calories**: 249

- **Protein Count**: 38 g

- **Fat Content**: 4 g

- **Carbs**: 11 g

List of Ingredients Needed:

- Chicken broth (.25 cup)

- Liquid aminos or soy sauce (.25 cup)

- Rice vinegar (.25 cup)

- Honey (6 tsp.)

- Ginger (1 tbsp.)

- Crushed red peppers (1 tsp.)

- Garlic (2 cloves)

- Orange Juice & zest (1 whole orange)

- Chicken breast partially frozen (1.5 lb.)

- Arrowroot powder (2 tsp.)

Preparation Technique:

1. Mince the garlic and dice the peppers. Juice and zest the orange. Dice the chicken into one-inch cubes.

2. Warm the Instant Pot using the sauté mode. Mix the broth, honey, aminos, vinegar, ginger, garlic, red peppers, orange zest, and orange juice.

3. When the orange sauce starts to boil, toss in the chicken breast chunks. Stir to coat the chicken.

4. Securely close the lid and set the timer for seven minutes using the high-pressure mode. Fully defrosted chicken will need to cook for five minutes.

5. When it's done cooking, natural-release the steam pressure (10 min.).

6. Remove the lid from the pot. Scoop up some of the sauce to make a slurry. Whisk the arrowroot powder/baking soda into the sauce in the measuring cup, then mix the thickened sauce back into the Instant Pot.

7. Rewarm the sauce again for it to thicken.

8. Serve the orange chicken in a large serving bowl over brown rice with grilled veggies on the side.

Rotisserie Chicken

Serving Yields: 6

Points Allotted - Smart Points: 6

Prep & Cooking Time: 50 minutes

Nutritional Macros Per Serving:

- **Calories**: 223

- **Protein Count**: 30 g

- **Fat Content**: 8 g

- **Carbs**: 1 g

List of Ingredients Needed:

- Whole chicken (4 lb.)

- Chicken broth - Fat-free or Water (1 cup)

- Paprika (.5 tbsp.)

- Pepper (1 tsp.)

- Salt (1.5 tsp.)

- Granulated garlic (.5 tbsp.)

- Onion powder (.5 tbsp.)

- Avocado/coconut oil (1.5 tbsp.)

Preparation Technique:

1. Discard the 'guts' from the chicken cavity and rinse it thoroughly, Dab it dry with paper towels.

2. Whisk the oil and spices in a small mixing bowl to make a paste. Rub the mixture over all parts of the chicken.

3. Warm the Instant Pot on using the sauté mode. When it's hot, arrange the chicken in the pot with the breast-side facing downward.

4. Sauté the breasts for about three to four minutes to brown and crisp the skin. Flip it over to sauté for another two to three minutes.

5. Pour in the chicken stock. Securely close the top and set the Instant Pot using the high-pressure function for 25 minutes. Natural-release the pressure (about 10-15 min.).

6. Take the top off of the pot and transfer chicken to a serving platter. Spoon some juices from the pot and serve as desired.

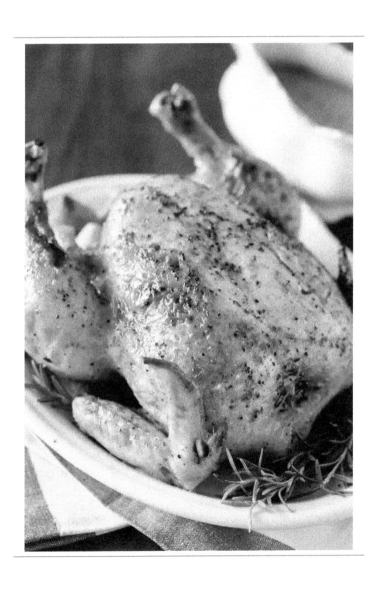

Salsa Chicken

Serving Yields: 6 = 1 cup salsa chicken + .5 cup rice

Points Allotted - Smart Points: 3

Prep & Cooking Time: 20 minutes

Nutritional Macros Per Serving:

- **Calories**: 332

- **Protein Count**: 23.8 g

- **Fat Content**: 10.7 g

- **Carbs**: 37.7 g

List of Ingredients Needed:

- Garlic cloves (1 tbsp.)

- Medium onion (1)

- Olive oil (1 tbsp.)

- Chicken breast (1 lb. boneless)

- Low-sodium chicken broth (.5 cup)

- Black beans (15 oz. can)

- Sweet corn (15 oz. can)

- Jar of salsa (1)

- Taco seasoning (1 packet)

- Uncle Ben's (preferred - 1 pouch)

Preparation Technique:

1. Drain and rinse the black beans and corn.

2. Heat the oil in the Instant Pot using the sauté function. Mince/chop the garlic and onion.

3. Once it's hot, toss in the onions and garlic. Sauté until the onion is translucent.

4. Mix in the chicken and sprinkle the package of taco seasoning over the breasts.

5. Stir in the salsa, corn, and black beans into the Instant Pot.

6. Use the manual mode for cooking the salsa chicken using the high-pressure setting for ten minutes.

7. Quick-release the built-up steam pressure, or wait and use the natural release (10 min.).

8. Once the Instant Pot is finished cooking, take the chicken out and shred it.

9. Toss it back into the Instant Pot and stir to serve immediately over rice or in taco shells.

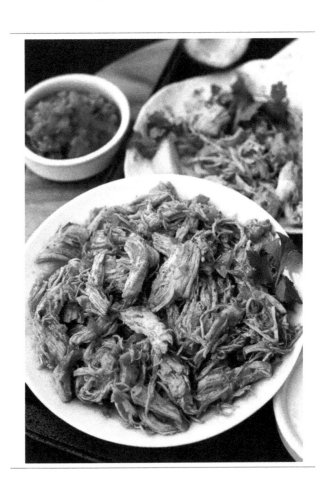

Spaghetti Squash Chicken Alfredo

Serving Yields: 5

Points Allotted - Smart Points: 15

Prep & Cooking Time: 40 minutes

Nutritional Macros Per Serving:

- **Calories**: 299
- **Protein Count**: 10 g
- **Fat Content**: 24 g
- **Carbs**: 9 g

List of Ingredients Needed:

- Spaghetti squash (1 whole)
- Skinless chicken breasts (16 oz. in cubes)
- Reduced-fat cream (4 oz.)
- Low-salt chicken broth (.5 cup)
- Chopped broccoli (2 cups)
- Parmesan cheese (1 cup)
- Heavy whipping cream (.25 cup)
- Unchilled butter (.75 tbsp.)
- Flour (1 tbsp.)
- Minced garlic (1 tbsp.)
- Almond milk (2 cups)
- Water (1 cup)
- Olive oil (1 tsp.)

Preparation Technique:

1. Use a sharp knife to slice the squash in half and discard the seeds.

2. Pour a cup of water in the pot. Add the trivet with the squash.

3. Securely close the lid and set the timer for 7 minutes using high pressure. Quick-release the steam and remove the squash. Shred it with a fork.

4. Dot the chicken with the seasonings. Add the oil to the Instant Pot.

5. Sauté the bird until done. Toss in the minced garlic while it's cooking.

6. Pour in the milk, whipping cream butter and cheese. Mix it all together and sauté for two to three minutes until the chopped broccoli is tender (or toss into a food processor).

7. Serve with the cream sauce and spaghetti squash.

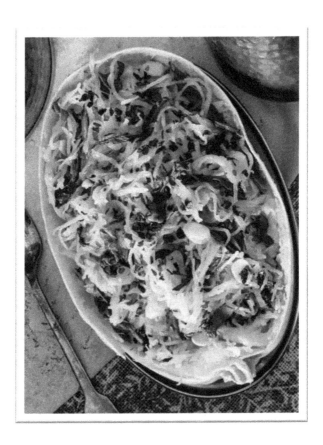

Spaghetti With Meat Sauce

Serving Yields: 5

Points Allotted - Smart Points:

Green: 10/Blue: 11/ Purple: 6

Prep & Cooking Time: 30 minutes

Nutritional Macros Per Serving:

- **Calories**: 390

- **Protein Count**: 23.5 g

- **Fat Content**: 14 g

- **Carbs**: 44 g

List of Ingredients Needed:

- 93% ground turkey (1 lb.)

- Kosher salt (.75 tsp.)

- Onion (.25 cup)

- Garlic (1 clove)

- Delallo Tomato Basil Pomodoro Sauce (1 jar, 25.25 oz.)

- Water (2 cups)

- Whole wheat or gluten-free spaghetti (8 oz.)

- Optional: Grated parmesan cheese - for serving

Preparation Technique:

1. Select the sauté function on the Instant Pot. When it's hot, add the turkey and salt. Sauté it for about three minutes.

2. Dice and toss in the onions and garlic. Sauté it until softened for 3 to 4 minutes.

3. Add the Pomodoro sauce, water, and spaghetti (broken in half), making sure the liquid covers everything without stirring.

4. Securely close the lid and set the Instant Pot on high pressure for 9 minutes.

5. Quick-release the pressure when it's done, so the pasta doesn't continue cooking.

6. Serve it topped with grated cheese if desired.

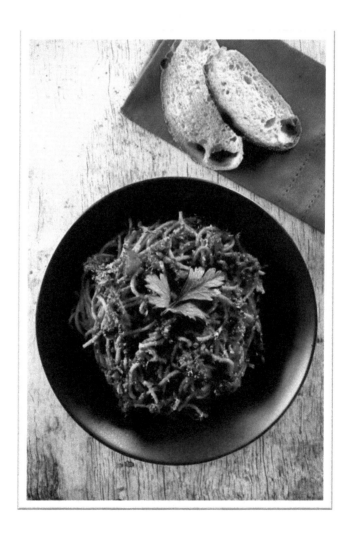

Sweet & Sour Chicken

Serving Yields: 8

Points Allotted - Smart Points: 0

Prep & Cooking Time: 30 minutes

Nutritional Macros Per Serving:

- **Calories**: 274

- **Protein Count**: 39 g

- **Fat Content**: 2 g

- **Carbs**: 12 g

List of Ingredients Needed:

- Chicken breasts (3 lb.)

- Pineapple (12 oz. jar)

- Pineapple salsa (16 oz. jar)

- Red pepper (1)

- Green pepper (1)

- Water (.5 cup)

- Salt (1 tsp.)

Preparation Technique:

1. Coat the bottom of the Instant Pot using a non-stick cooking spray.

2. Cut the skin and bones from the chicken.

3. Using the sauté setting, brown the chicken on all sides (3-4 minutes).

4. Chop the pineapple and peppers. Add the rest of the fixings into the pot. Select the high setting for 12 minutes.

5. Use a quick-release of pressure, then cut the chicken into smaller chunks or slices.

6. It can be served over rice if desired.

Sweet & Spicy BBQ Chicken Wings

Serving Yields: 6

Points Allotted - Smart Points: 13

Prep & Cooking Time: 35 minutes

Nutritional Macros Per Serving:

- **Calories**: 321

- **Protein Count**: 27.2 g

- **Fat Content**: 19.5 g

- **Carbs**: 7.3 g

List of Ingredients Needed:

- Frank's Red Hot Sauce (.25 cup)

- Tomato paste (4 oz.)

- Liquid smoke (1 tsp.)

- Apple cider vinegar (.5 cup)

- Water (.5 cup)

- Ground Cayenne pepper (.125 tsp.)

- Chipotle Chile - ground (.125 tsp.)

- Crushed red pepper flakes (.25 tsp.)

- Cinnamon (1 tsp.)

- Paprika (.5 tsp.)

- Salt (1 tsp.)

- Golden monk fruit sweetener (2.5 tbsp.)

For the Wings:

- Chicken wings (2 lb.)

- Coarse salt (1 tbsp.)

Preparation Technique:

1. Toss all of the sauce ingredients into the Instant Pot using the sauté function for about ten minutes.

2. Add in the wings and salt to the cooker.

3. Securely close the lid and set the timer for ten minutes using high pressure.

4. Quick-release the pressure and open the pot.

5. Rotate the wings and brush the sauce over the wings. Set the cooker for another ten minutes under high pressure until done. Serve.

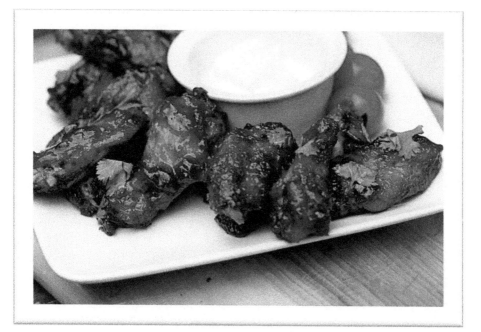

Teriyaki Meatballs

Serving Yields: 7 - 2 each serving

Points Allotted - Smart Points: 8

Prep & Cooking Time: 30 minutes

Nutritional Macros Per Serving:

- **Calories**: 261

- **Protein Count**: 34 g

- **Fat Content**: 5 g

- **Carbs**: 20 g

List of Ingredients Needed:

- Ground turkey (2 lb.)

- Eggs (2)

- Ground ginger (1 tsp.)

- Aminos or low sodium soy sauce (1 tsp.)

- Rolled oats (.5 cup)

- Garlic (1 tbsp.)

- Chopped green onions (.5 cup)

The Rice:

- Brown rice (1.5 cups)

- Water (2 cups)

The Glaze:

- Aminos (2 tbsp.)

- Water (.25 cup)

- Vinegar (1 tsp.)

- Honey (1 tbsp.)

- Ginger (.5 tsp.)

Preparation Technique:

1. Mince the garlic and combine all the fixings for the meatballs in a large mixing container.

2. Fill the silicone egg bite molds with the meatball mixture. Cover the meatballs with foil or a silicone food cover and place them on a trivet with long handles.

3. Add two cups of water and the brown rice to the Instant Pot insert.

4. Arrange the trivet/basket with the meatballs over the rice.

5. Note: (If you are not cooking rice with the meatballs, then just add the water to the bottom of the Instant Pot insert.)

6. Secure the lid and set the Instant Pot using the high-pressure setting for 25 minutes. Natural-release the pressure for about 10 minutes once the buzzer goes off.

7. While the pressure is releasing, pour the water into a skillet using the med-high temperature setting. When the water starts to simmer, stir in the aminos, honey, and ginger.

8. Wait for it to boil, then pour in the vinegar.

9. Turn the burner to med-low. Stir the glaze while the water evaporates, and the glaze thickens. When the sauce is thickened, remove it from the heat until you're ready to coat the meatballs.

10. Add and roll the meatballs in the glaze until they are all lightly coated. Serve the meatballs over rice with a side of steamed veggies.

Tikka Masala

Serving Yields: 6

Points Allotted - Smart Points:

Green: 6/Blue: 3/ Purple: 3

Prep & Cooking Time:
30 minutes

Nutritional Macros Per Serving:

- **Calories**: 301

- **Protein Count**: 35 g

- **Fat Content**: 11 g

- **Carbs**: 13 g

List of Ingredients Needed:

- Chicken breast (2 lbs. boneless - skinless)

- Coconut oil (1 tsp.)

- Large onion (1)

- Cloves of garlic (4)

- Ginger (1 tbsp.)

- Garam masala (2 tbsp.)

- Paprika (2 tsp.)

- Canned fire-roasted diced tomatoes (28 oz.)

- Canned coconut milk (.75 cup)

- Kosher salt (2 tsp.)

- Cilantro (.33 cup)

Preparation Technique:

1. Warm the Instant Pot using the sauté mode. Pour in the coconut oil to melt.

2. Mince the garlic and grate the ginger. Chop the cilantro.

3. Once the oil is melted, toss in the onion, garlic, ginger, garam masala, paprika, and salt. Sauté the mixture for four to five minutes until the onions have softened.

4. Turn off the sauté function. Pour in
   scrape any browned bits off the bott
   the chicken.

5. Close the Instant Pot and choose the Poultry setting for
   15 minutes. Natural-release the pressure for ten
   minutes.

6. Carefully open the lid, and s

7. Taste it and adjust the seas
   using the cilantro as a garni

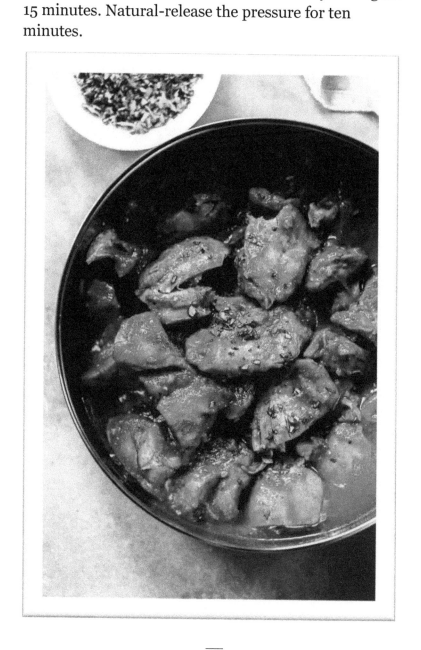

Turkey Meatball Stroganoff

Serving Yields: 4

Points Allotted - Smart Points:

Green: 7/Blue: 7/ Purple: 7

Prep & Cooking Time: 40 minutes

Nutritional Macros Per Serving: 5 each serving:

- **Calories**: 310

- **Protein Count**: 27.5 g

- **Fat Content**: 16 g

- **Carbs**: 14.5 g

List of Ingredients Needed:

- Olive oil, divided (1 tsp.)

- Chopped onion (.5 cup)

- 93% ground turkey (1 lb.)

- Whole wheat seasoned breadcrumbs (.33 cup)

- Egg (1 large)

- Chopped parsley (.25 cup - divided)

- Fat-free milk (3 tbsp.)

- Kosher salt (.75 tsp.)

- Black pepper (as desired)

- Water (.75 cup)

- Light sour cream (.5 cup)

- All-purpose flour (2 tbsp.)

- Tomato paste (2 tsp.)

- Beef Bouillon - ex. Better Than Bouillon (2 tsp.)

- Worcestershire sauce (.5 tsp.)

- Paprika (.5 tsp.)

- Sliced Cremini mushrooms (8 oz.)

- Fresh thyme (1 sprig)

Preparation Technique:

1. Warm the Instant Pot using the sauté function. Lightly spritz it with a cooking oil spray.

2. Mince and add the onions to the cooker to sauté for two to three minutes. Remove them from the cooker and divide them into two portions.

3. Combine half of the sautéed onions with the turkey, breadcrumbs, milk, egg, two tablespoons of parsley, black pepper, and ¾ teaspoons of salt. Shape the prepared mixture into about 20 meatballs.

4. In a blender, combine the sour cream, water, flour, bouillon, Worcestershire sauce, tomato paste, and paprika. Blend the mixture thoroughly.

5. Heat the Instant Pot using the sauté mode, and pour in the oil.

6. Sauté half of the meatballs without disturbing for about two minutes and set them aside on a platter. Repeat with remaining meatballs.

7. Place all the meatballs, the rest of the onions, and sauce over the meatballs. Mix in the mushrooms and thyme into the Instant Pot.

8. Set the cooker using the high-pressure setting for 10 minutes.

9. Natural-release the pressure. After about ten minutes, open the lid and garnish it with additional thyme, parsley, if desired before serving over your favorite noodles.

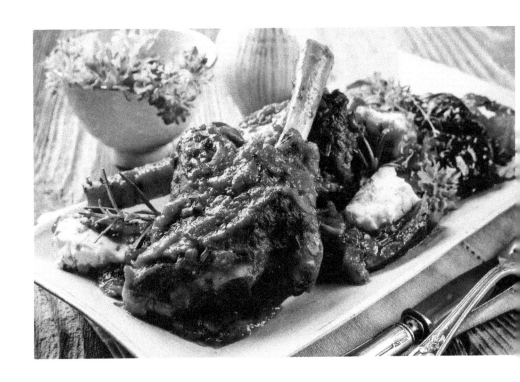

Italian Pulled Pork

Serving Yields: 10

Points Allotted - Smart Points:

Green: 1/Blue: 1/ Purple: 1

Prep & Cooking Time: 1 hour 10 minutes

Nutritional Macros Per Serving:

- **Calories**: 93

- **Protein Count**: 11 g

- **Fat Content**: 1.5 g

- **Carbs**: 6.5 g

List of Ingredients Needed:

- Pork tenderloin (18 oz.)

- Black pepper (as desired)

- Kosher salt (1 tsp.)

- Olive oil (1 tsp.)

- Cloves of garlic (5 smashed with the side of a knife)

- Crushed tomatoes - ex. Tuttorosso (28 oz. can)

- Roasted red peppers - drained (7 oz. jar)

- Fresh thyme (2 sprigs)

- Bay leaves (2)

- Chopped fresh parsley - divided (1 tbsp.)

Preparation Technique:

1. Sprinkle the meat using the black pepper and salt.

2. Select the sauté mode and pour in the oil to warm the Instant Pot. Mince and toss in the garlic to sauté it until golden brown (1-1.5 minutes). Transfer them from the pot with a slotted spoon.

3. Mix in the pork and sauté for about two minutes per side. Add the rest of the fixings (and garlic), reserving half of the parsley.

4. Set the cooker using the high-pressure setting for 45 minutes.

5. When it's done, merely natural-release the pressure. Remove the bay leaves, shred the pork, and top with the rest of the parsley. Serve the tasty pulled pork over your favorite pasta.

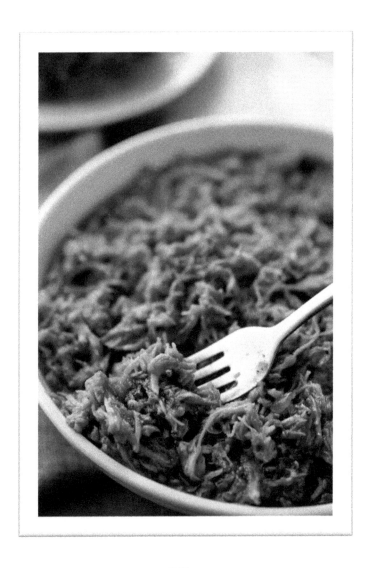

Mu Shu Pork Tacos

Serving Yields: 8

Points Allotted - Smart Points: 3

Prep & Cooking Time: 35 minutes

Nutritional Macros Per Serving:

- **Calories**: 164

- **Protein Count**: 15 g

- **Fat Content**: 8 g

- **Carbs**: 6 g

List of Ingredients Needed:

- Thinly sliced boneless pork chops (1 lb.)

- Cabbage/ lettuce – divided (.5 of 1 head)

- Toasted sesame oil – divided (2 tbsp.)

- Low-sodium soy sauce/Bragg Liquid Aminos (3 tbsp.)

- Hoisin sauce (1 tbsp.)

- Matchstick carrots (.5 cup)

- Minced garlic (1 tbsp.)

- White mushrooms (3 cups)

- Green onions (1 cup)

- Cornstarch (1 tbsp.)

- Water (4 tbsp.)

Preparation Technique:

1. Remove eight leaves of cabbage or lettuce and set them aside for the tortillas. Chop the remainder of cabbage, mushrooms, and green onions, and place them aside for now.

2. Combine the hoisin and soy sauce with the pork, one tablespoon of sesame oil, and cornstarch.

3. Use the sauté mode and add one tablespoon of the oil and garlic to the Instant Pot. Sauté for about three minutes, and mix in the pork mixture and water.

4. Once it starts to brown, add the chopped cabbage, carrots, water, and mushrooms. Secure the lid and cook for 15 minutes.

5. Serve with one cup of the mu shu pork on a leaf of cabbage and serve.

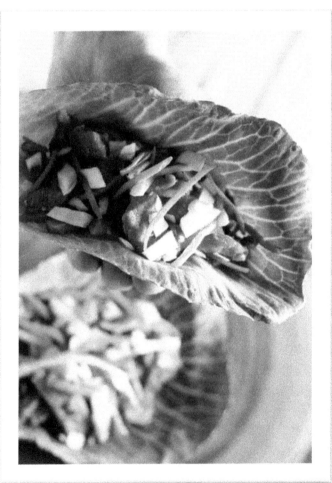

Sausage Cabbage Bowl with Quinoa

Serving Yields: 6

Points Allotted - Smart Points: 5

Prep & Cooking Time: 52 minutes

Nutritional Macros Per Serving:

- **Calories**: 233
- **Protein Count**: 16.7 g
- **Fat Content**: 8.9 g
- **Carbs**: 26 g

List of Ingredients Needed:

- Olive oil (2 tsp.)
- Raw hot or sweet Italian chicken sausage (1 lb.)
- Chopped yellow onion (1)
- Garlic cloves (3)
- Paprika (1 tsp.)
- Dried oregano (1 tsp.)
- Salt (.75 tsp.)
- Low-sodium chicken broth (1.25 cup)
- Ground pepper (.5 tsp.)
- Canned petite diced tomatoes (1 cup)
- Dry quinoa (.5 cup)
- Thinly sliced cabbage (About 12 cups/1.75 lb.)
- Minced Italian parsley (.25 cup)

Preparation Technique:

1. Set the Instant Pot using the sauté function, adding the oil to heat.

2. Add the chicken sausage (squeezed out of casings) and onion, and cook, breaking up the sausage until its browned or about five minutes. Mix in the paprika, garlic, oregano, pepper, and salt.

3. Pour in the diced tomatoes and broth. Securely close the lid and cook for 12 minutes (high-pressure).

4. When it buzzes, quick-release the built-up steam and stir in the quinoa.

5. Toss in the cabbage, but do NOT stir. Securely close the top and set it on high pressure to three minutes. Quick-release the steam and sprinkle it with parsley before serving.

Sweet Cranberry Pork

Serving Yields: 3

Points Allotted - Smart Points: 6

Prep & Cooking Time: 30-35 minutes

Nutritional Macros Per Serving:

- **Calories**: 202

- **Protein Count**: 18.5 g

- **Fat Content**: 11 g

- **Carbs**: 4 g

List of Ingredients Needed:

- Coconut oil (1 tbsp.)

- Cranberries (1 cup)

- Arugula (2 cups)

- Pork leg (7 oz.)

- Pine nuts (2 tbsp.)

- Lemon juice (1 tbsp.)

- Nutmeg (.25 tsp.)

- Coconut sugar (1 tsp.)

Preparation Technique:

1. Add the berries to the Instant Pot in enough water to cover. Stir in the nutmeg and sugar.

2. Secure the top and set for three minutes using high-pressure.

3. Natural-release the steam and transfer the berries to a deep mixing container.

4. Choose the sauté function to melt the oil. Stir in the pine nuts and sauté for about two to three minutes as needed. Mix in the meat and cook for another five to six minutes.

5. Stir in the cranberry sauce and let it boil. When it's hot, divide into three portions and add the arugula. Drizzle with lemon juice and serve.

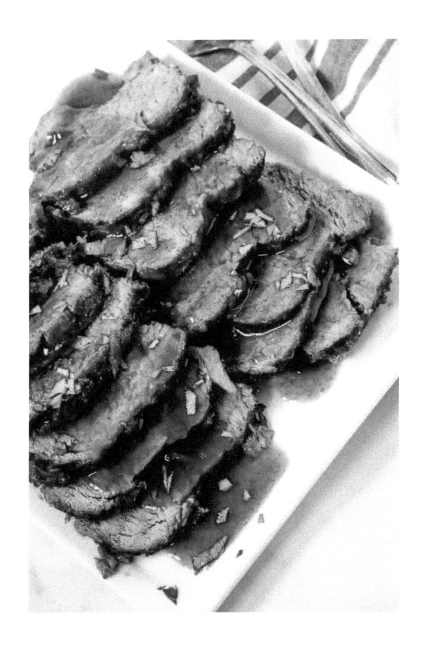

Moroccan Meatballs

Serving Yields: 4

Points Allotted - Smart Points: 4

Green: /Blue: / Purple: /Old Plan:

Prep & Cooking Time: 30-35 minutes

Nutritional Macros Per Serving:

- **Calories**: 307
- **Protein Count**: 33 g
- **Fat Content**: 12.3 g
- **Carbs**: 15.4 g

List of Ingredients Needed:

The Meatballs:

- 95/5 extra-lean ground beef (1 lb. . .)
- Onion (1 small)
- Cloves of garlic (4)
- Cumin (1 tbsp.)
- Smoked paprika (1 tsp.)
- Ground coriander (1 tsp.)
- Allspice (.5 tsp.)
- Salt and pepper to taste
- Fresh cilantro (2 tbsp.)
- Fresh parsley (2 tbsp.)

The Sauce:

- Diced tomatoes (23 oz. can)
- Small onion (1)
- Pitted green olives (.5 cup)
- Tomato paste (1 tbsp.)
- Cumin (2 tsp.)
- Garlic (2 cloves)
- Turmeric (1 tsp.)
- Paprika (1 tsp.)
- Salt and pepper (as desired)

Preparation Technique:

1. Set the Instant Pot to the sauté function. Finely chop the olives, parsley, and cilantro.

2. When the pot is hot, mist it lightly with oil. Mince the onions and garlic.

3. Add in the onions (from the sauce ingredients) and sauté them for about three to four minutes.

4. Stir in the remaining sauce ingredients and mix well.

5. Place the meatballs into the sauce, cover, and cook using high pressure for 15 minutes. Natural-release the pressure for 10 minutes, open the lid, and serve.

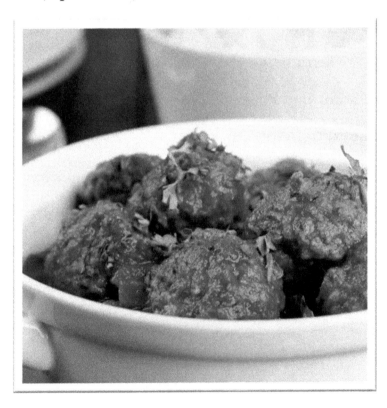

Picadillo – American/Latin/Cuban Cuisine

Serving Yields: 6/0.5 cup each

Points Allotted - Smart Points:

Green: 2/Blue: 3/ Purple: 4

Prep & Cooking Time: 25 minutes

Nutritional Macros Per Serving:

- **Calories**: 207

- **Protein Count**: 25 g

- **Fat Content**: 8.5 g

- **Carbs**: 5 g

List of Ingredients Needed:

- 93% lean ground beef (1.5 lb.)

- Chopped onion (half of 1 large)

- Cloves of garlic (2 minced)

- Tomato (1 chopped)

- Red bell pepper (half of 1)

- Cilantro (2 tbsp.)

- Kosher salt (1 tsp.)

- Tomato sauce - ex. Goya (half of a 4 oz. can)

- Ground cumin (1 tsp.)

- Bay leaf (1-2)

- Capers or green olives (2 tbsp.)

Preparation Technique:

1. Select the sauté function to heat the Instant Pot.

2. Brown the meat with a portion of salt and pepper, cooking until it's no longer pink.

3. Finely chop the bell pepper. Mix in the garlic, onion, salt, peppers, tomato, and cilantro. Stir for one minute, and add the capers/olives with about two tablespoons of the brine (the juice from the olives), bay leaf, and cumin.

4. Pour in the tomato sauce and three tablespoons of water, mixing thoroughly.

5. Securely close the top and set it using the high-pressure setting (15 min.). Natural-release the steam and serve.

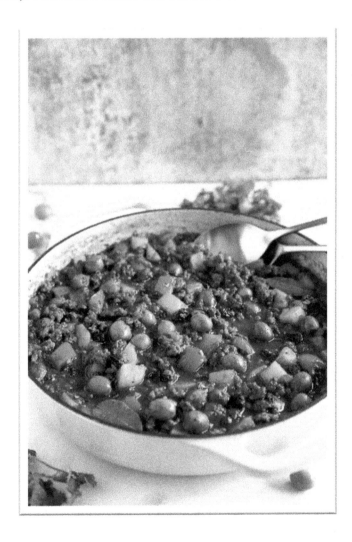

Sesame Beef

Serving Yields: 6

Points Allotted - Smart Points:

Green: 5/Blue: 5/ Purple: 5

Prep & Cooking Time: 1 hour 10 minutes

Nutritional Macros Per Serving:

- **Calories**: 254

- **Protein Count**: 36 g

- **Fat Content**: 7 g

- **Carbs**: 10 g

List of Ingredients Needed:

- Unsweetened applesauce (.5 cup)

- Soy sauce or coconut aminos (.25 cup)

- Brown sugar or honey (2 tbsp.)

- Garlic (2 cloves)

- Grated ginger (.5 tbsp.)

- Toasted sesame oil (2 tsp.)

- Lean beef eye round roast (2 lb.)

- Cornstarch (1 tbsp.)

- Sesame seeds (1 tbsp.)

Preparation Technique:

1. Add the beef to the Instant Pot with all of the sauce fixings. Cover and set the Manual timer to 45 minutes using high pressure.

2. Once it is cooked, you can manually release or naturally release the steam. Use two forks to shred the beef. If the sauce is liquidly, combine the cornstarch with 1-2 tablespoons of

cold water until it
dissolves.

3. Add it to the pot along with the beef and turn the Instant Pot to
   the sauté mode. Wait for the sauce to come to a simmer, and
   then turn off the heat.

4. Let the meat rest for a few minutes so the sauce can thicken.

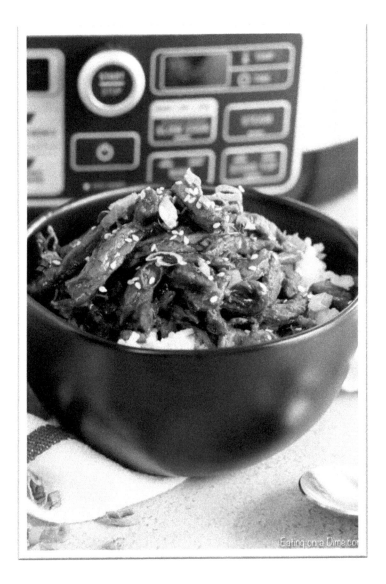

Sunday Pot Roast

Serving Yields: 8

Points Allotted - Smart Points: 7

Prep & Cooking Time: 1 hour 45 minutes

Nutritional Macros Per Serving:

- **Calories**: 389

- **Protein Count**: 48 g

- **Fat Content**: 13 g

- **Carbs**: 20 g

List of Ingredients Needed:

- Beef chuck roast (3 lb. - fat trimmed)

- Olive oil (1 tbsp.)

- Onion soup mix (2 packets)

- Large onion (1 - roughly chopped)

- Worcestershire sauce (3 tbsp.)

- Fat-free beef broth (1.5 cups)

- Large carrots (3 - cut into large chunks)

- Yukon gold potatoes (1 lb.)

- Salt and pepper (to your liking)

Preparation Technique:

1. Sprinkle both sides of the roast with black pepper and salt. Whisk the onion soup mix, broth, and Worcestershire sauce.

2. Add the oil and warm the Instant Pot using the sauté mode. When it's hot, add in the meat and sauté it for about one to two minutes on each side.

3. Cut the potatoes into large chunks. Top the meat with potatoes, onions, and carrots, and the prepared sauce.

4. Turn off the sauté function

5. Securely close the top and set the timer for 70 minutes using the high-pressure setting.

6. Natural-release the pressure (10 min.), then quick-release the rest of the steam pressure.

7. Transfer the roast from the pot and shred to your liking. Serve with the veggies.

Unstuffed Cabbage Bowls

Serving Yields: 4/1.5 cups each

Points Allotted - Smart Points:

Green: 8/Blue: 8/ Purple: 6

Prep & Cooking Time: 30 minutes

Nutritional Macros Per Serving:

- **Calories**: 338

- **Protein Count**: 30.5 g

- **Fat Content**: 8 g

- **Carbs**: 36 g

List of Ingredients Needed:

- Lean - 93% - ground beef (1 lb.)

- Chopped onion (1 cup)

- Garlic (1 minced clove)

- Kosher salt (1.25 tsp.)

- Dried marjoram (1 tbsp.)

- Black pepper (as desired)

- Tomato sauce (8 oz. can)

- Hungarian paprika (.5 tsp.)

- Low-sodium beef broth (1 cup)

- Raisins (2 tbsp.)

- Cooked brown rice (1 cup)

- Medium head cabbage - cored and chopped (1 head or 9 cups)

Seafood Options

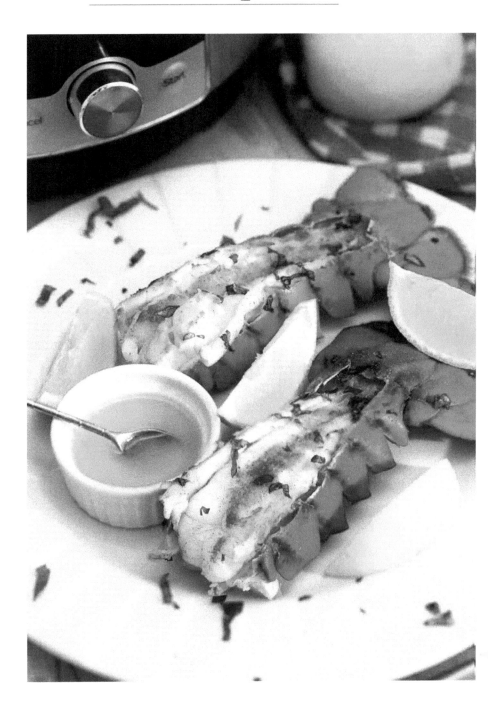

Anchovies & Buttery Rosemary Sauce

Serving Yields: 3-4

Points Allotted - Smart Points: 5

Prep & Cooking Time: 18-20 minutes

Nutritional Macros Per Serving:

- **Calories**: 327
- **Protein Count**: 28 g
- **Fat Content**: 24.5 g
- **Carbs**: 4.5 g

List of Ingredients Needed:

- Anchovies (10 oz.)
- Butter (4 tbsp.)
- Sea salt (1 tsp.)
- Paprika (.5 tsp.)
- Red chili pepper (1 - seeded & sliced)
- Rosemary (1 tsp.)
- Dried dill (1 tsp.)
- Basil (1 tbsp.)
- Red chili flakes (1 tsp.)
- Breadcrumbs (.33 cup)

Preparation Technique:

1. Whisk the rosemary, dill, basil, salt, paprika, and chili flakes. Cover the anchovies with the spices. Add in the chili pepper and wait for about ten minutes while it marinates.

2. Warm the Instant Pot using the sauté function and add the butter.

3. Dip the anchovies in the breadcrumbs and add them to the pot.

4. Sauté the anchovies four minutes per side and drain on paper towels before serving.

Banana Mackerel

Serving Yields: 5

Points Allotted - Smart Points: 6

Prep & Cooking Time: 38-40 minutes

Nutritional Macros Per Serving:

- **Calories**: 196

- **Protein Count**: 21 g

- **Fat Content**: 5.5 g

- **Carbs**: 18 g

List of Ingredients Needed:

- Water (2 tbsp. + .25 cup)

- Olive oil (1 tsp.)

- Cream (.25 cup)

- Ripe bananas (3)

- Brown sugar (1 tsp.)

- Oregano (3 tbsp.)

- Mackerel (1 lb.)

- Ground white pepper (1tsp.)

- Cinnamon (.25 tsp.)

Preparation Technique:

1. Peel and chop the bananas. Sprinkle with sugar and add the cream, mixing well.

2. Heat the Instant Pot using the sauté mode.

3. Mix in the banana mixture and sauté for 8 minutes. Stir often.

4. Chop and mix the fish, pepper, water, oil, and cinnamon.

5. Combine all of the fixings in the cooker and securely close the lid.

6.   Make sure the valve is sealed and set the timer for 20 minutes using the Meat/Stew function.

7.   When the time has elapsed, quick-release the steam pressure, open the top, and serve the delicious fish dish.

Bang Bang Shrimp Pasta

Serving Yields: 6

Points Allotted - Smart Points: 12

Prep & Cooking Time: 11 minutes

Nutritional Macros Per Serving:

- **Calories**: 501

- **Protein Count**: 25 g

- **Fat Content**: 9g

- **Carbs**: 76 g

List of Ingredients Needed:

- Dried spaghetti (1 lb.)

- Garlic (3 cloves)

- Coconut oil (1 tsp.)

- Water (4.25 cups)

- Jumbo raw shrimp (1 lb.)

- Light mayo (.75 cup)

- Thai sweet chili sauce (.75 cup)

- Sriracha sauce (1 tbsp.)

- Lime juice (.25 cup)

- Chopped scallions (.5 cup)

- Pepper and salt (to taste)

Preparation Technique:

1. Mince and mix the garlic, oil, water, and about one teaspoon of salt.

2. Add this to the Instant Pot and set the timer at four minutes using the high-temperature setting.

3. When done, quick-release the pressure and open the lid.

4. Whisk the mayo, Thai sauce, juice, and sriracha. Add it to the pasta and mix it all with the scallions, and shrimp in the Instant Pot.

5. Sauté them for two to three minutes or until they turn pink. Season them as desired and serve right away.

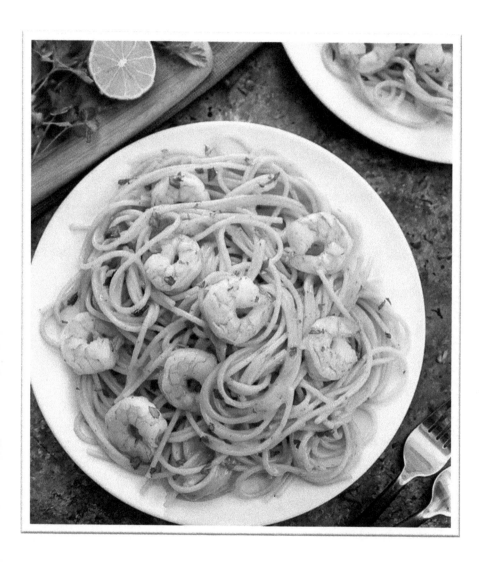

Cajun Shrimp & Sausage Boil

Serving Yields: 5

Points Allotted - Smart Points: 9

Prep & Cooking Time: 20 minutes

Nutritional Macros Per Serving:

- **Calories**: 514

- **Protein Count**: 38 g

- **Fat Content**: 35 g

- **Carbs**: 9 g

List of Ingredients Needed:

- Smoked sausage (.5 lb.)

- Corn (4 ears)

- Red potatoes (2 halved)

- Louisiana Shrimp & Crab Boil (1 tbsp.)

- Water to cover above toppings (as needed)

- Raw shrimp (.5 lb.)

The Sauce:

- Butter (6 tbsp.)

- Minced garlic (1 tbsp.)

- Cajun seasoning (.125 tsp.)

- Old Bay Seasoning (.25 tsp.)

- Louisiana Hot Sauce (3-5 shakes/as desired)

- Lemon pepper (.125 tsp.)

- Juiced lemon (half of 1)

Preparation Technique:

1. Add the sausage, corn, and potatoes to the Instant Pot, adding the water and boil mix. Set the timer on the cooker for four minutes.

2. Dissolve the butter using the med-high temperature setting on the stovetop. Toss in the garlic to sauté with the rest of the seasonings.

3. When done, quick-release the pressure on the Instant Pot and open the lid.

4. Add everything together and serve right away for the best results.

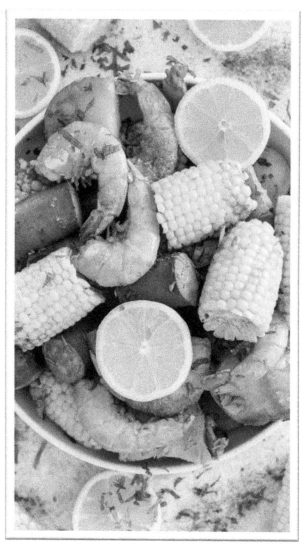

Crustless Crab Quiche

Serving Yields: 4

Points Allotted - Smart Points: 13

Prep & Cooking Time: 60 minutes

Nutritional Macros Per Serving:

- **Calories**: 395

- **Protein Count**: 22 g

- **Fat Content**: 25 g

- **Carbs**: 19 g

List of Ingredients Needed:

- Eggs (4)

- Half & Half (1 cup)

- Black pepper (1 tsp.)

- Salt (.5 to 1 tsp.)

- Herbes de Provence (1 tsp.)

- Smoked paprika (1 tsp.)

- Green onions (1 cup - chopped)

- Shredded parmesan (1 cup)

- Real crabmeat (8 oz.)

- Imitation crabmeat (8 oz.)

Preparation Technique:

1. Whisk the creamer, salt, pepper, paprika, Herbes de Provence, and eggs in a large mixing container.

2. Mix in the onions and crabmeat in a heatproof dish to add to the Instant Pot.

3. Pour some water into the cooker and add the steamer rack/trivet.

4. Place the bowl on the rack and set the timer on high for 40 minutes.

5. Natural-release the pressure for about ten minutes and open the lid to serve.

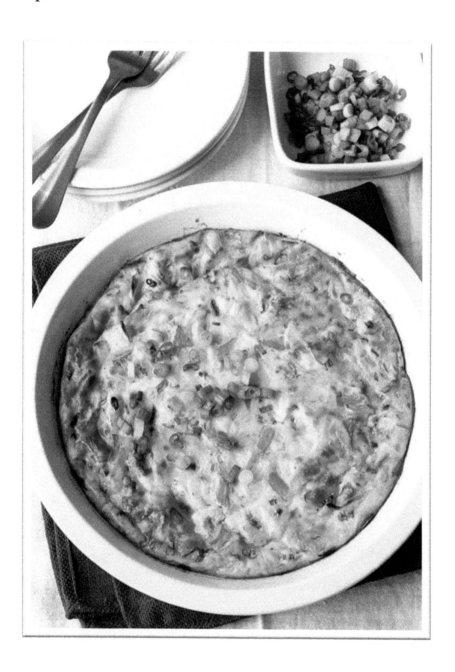

Drunken Clams

Serving Yields: 6

Points Allotted - Smart Points: 17

Prep & Cooking Time: 30 minutes

Nutritional Macros Per Serving:

- **Calories**: 455

- **Protein Count**: 32 g

- **Fat Content**: 21 g

- **Carbs**: 14 g

List of Ingredients Needed:

- Olive oil (.25 cup)

- Garlic (2 cloves)

- Finely chopped basil (.25 cup)

- Pale ale (2 cups)

- Water (1 cup)

- Chicken broth (.5 cup)

- Dry white wine (.25 cup)

- Fresh clams (3 lb.)

- Fresh lemon juice (2 tbsp.)

Preparation Technique:

1. Warm the oil in the Instant Pot using the sauté function. Mince and add the garlic to sauté for two minutes.

2. Chop the basil and add it in with the broth, water, lager, wine, and lemon juice. Sauté for one minute.

3. Add the trivet/steamer basket and add the clams on it. Close the top and set the timer for four minutes using the high-pressure setting.

4. Quick-release the pressure and discard the unopened shells.

5. Place them in a bowl and serve with some of the cooking juices if desired.

Fish Tacos

Serving Yields: 4

Points Allotted - Smart Points: 7

Prep & Cooking Time: 25 minutes

Nutritional Macros Per Serving:

- **Calories**: 269

- **Protein Count**: 27 g

- **Fat Content**: 12 g

- **Carbs**: 18 g

List of Ingredients Needed:

- Tilapia fillets (2)

- Canola oil (1 tsp.)

- Smoked paprika (2 tbsp.)

- Salt (1 pinch)

- Lime juice (1 lime)

- Fresh cilantro (1-2 sprigs)

Preparation Technique:

1. Prepare the tilapia on a sheet of parchment paper or foil and coat it in the oil, paprika, salt, a spritz of lime, and cilantro.

2. Add a half cup of water to the pot and add the trivet. Add the bundled salmon on the trivet and set the timer for 8 minutes (high).

3. Make the tacos to your liking.

Herbed Salmon

Serving Yields: 4

Points Allotted - Smart Points: 1

Prep & Cooking Time: 20 minutes

Nutritional Macros Per Serving:

- **Calories**: 276
- **Protein Count**: 36.5 g
- **Fat Content**: 12.5 g
- **Carbs**: 6.5 g

List of Ingredients Needed:

- Chopped tomatoes (2)
- Dried basil (.5 tsp.)
- Rosemary (.25 tsp.)
- Oregano (.5 tsp.)
- Wild salmon (25 oz.)
- Pepper flakes (.25 tsp.)
- Balsamic vinegar (2 tbsp.)
- Freshly chopped basil (.25 cup)
- Salt & pepper (as desired)
- Olive oil (2 tsp.)
- Water (1 cup)

Preparation Technique:

1. Whisk the rosemary, salt, pepp pepper flakes, basil, and orega in a mixing dish. Season the salmon and place in foil.

2. Pour the water to the Instant P and place the trivet/steamer basket.

3. Place the salmon onto the rack and close the top (valve sealed

4. Adjust the timer for 8-10 minu using the manual function. Qu release when the timer buzzes.

5. Portion the salmon into the dishes.

6. Chop the basil and mix with the vinegar, tomatoes, oil, salt, and pepper. Set it aside and serve over the salmon.

Instant Pot Mussels

Serving Yields: 4

Points Allotted - Smart Points: 8

Prep & Cooking Time: 40 minutes

Nutritional Macros Per Serving:

- **Calories**: 189

- **Protein Count**: 14 g

- **Fat Content**: 8 g

- **Carbs**: 8 g

List of Ingredients Needed:

- Butter (2 tbsp.)

- Chopped shallots (2)

- Minced garlic (4 cloves)

- Broth (.5 cup)

- White wine (.5 cup)

- Cleaned mussels (2 lb.)

- For Serving: Optional: Lemon & Parsley

Preparation Technique:

1. Clean and remove the 'whiskers' from the mussels and discard the ones that do not close when tapped. Discard them if they have a split in them.

2. Prepare the Instant Pot using the sauté mode. Add the butter to melt.

3. Mince the onion and garlic and toss into the pot to sauté about one to two minutes, or until the onion is translucent.

4. Pour in the wine and soup.

5. Carefully add the mussels to the cooker and set the timer for five minutes. Natural-release the pressure for 10-15 minutes and open the lid.

6. Serve with a spritz of juice and dusting of parsley.

Salmon Broccoli & Potatoes

Serving Yields: 1

Points Allotted - Smart Points: 6

Prep & Cooking Time: 5 minutes

Nutritional Macros Per Serving:

- **Calories**: 384

- **Protein Count**: 35 g

- **Fat Content**: 18 g

- **Carbs**: 35 g

List of Ingredients Needed:

- Salmon fillet (72 g)

- Broccoli (70 g)

- New potatoes (250 g)

- Butter (1 tbsp.)

- Optional: Fresh herbs, salt, and pepper

Preparation Technique:

1. Rinse and chop the broccoli into small florets.

2. Pour ⅔ of a cup of water into the Instant Pot.

3. Season the potatoes with the chosen spices, adding them to the steamer rack/trivet. Spread butter over them and place them in the steamer for two minutes.

4. Quick-release the steam and place the salmon on the rack and cook another two minutes in the steamer mode.

5. Wait about 10-15 minutes and serve it warm.

Salmon & Vegetable Delight

Serving Yields: 4

Points Allotted - Smart Points: 2

Prep & Cooking Time: 18-20 minutes

Nutritional Macros Per Serving:

- **Calories**: 207

- **Protein Count**: 23 g

- **Fat Content**: 6.5 g

- **Carbs**: 8 g

List of Ingredients Needed:

- Olive oil (2 tsp.)

- Black pepper (3.5 tsp. or as desired)

- Salt (.25 tsp.)

- Water (.75 cup)

- Salmon fillet (1 lb. skin-on)

- Carrot (1)

- Bell pepper (1)

- Zucchini (1)

- Lemon slices (half of 1)

Preparation Technique:

1. Use a spiral slicer to julienne the pepper, carrot, and zucchini.

2. Coat the salmon with oil, salt, and pepper.

3. Open the Instant Pot to add the water and brivet. Add the salmon.

4. Quick-release the pressure and remove the salmon and rack.

5. Select the sauté mode and add the oil and veggies. Sauté for two minutes.

6. Serve the salmon and veggies.

Salmon With Orange Ginger Sauce

Serving Yields: 4

Points Allotted - Smart Points: 9

Prep & Cooking Time: 30 minutes

Nutritional Macros Per Serving:

- **Calories**: 166

- **Protein Count**: 23 g

- **Fat Content**: 7 g

- **Carbs**: 12 g

List of Ingredients Needed:

- Shrimp (1 lb.)

- Dark soy sauce (1 tbsp.)

- Minced ginger (2 tsp.)

- Minced garlic (1 tsp.)

- Ground black pepper (1 to 1.5 tsp.)

- Salt (1 tsp./as desired)

- Low-sugar marmalade (2 tsp.)

Preparation Technique:

1. Rinse and pat the salmon dry and put it into a 6-inch dish to place in the Instant Pot.

2. Whisk all of the fixings and pour them over the salmon to marinate for 15 to 30 minutes.

3. Add water and trivet into the Instant Pot.

4. Place the bowl and sauce on the rack and set the timer for three minutes on the low setting.

5. Natural-release the pressure for five minutes, and then quick-release the balance of it.

6. Serve as it is or sear it for three to four minutes or in the oven at 350° F until it's flaky.

Shrimp & Grits

Serving Yields: 4

Points Allotted - Smart Points: 8

Prep The & Cooking Time: 50 minutes

Nutritional Macros Per Serving:

- **Calories**: 292

- **Protein Count**: 30 g

- **Fat Content**: 9 g

- **Carbs**: 18 g

List of Ingredients Needed:

- Shrimp (1 lb.)

- Old Bay seasoning (2 tsp.)

- Diced strips of smoked bacon (3)

- Onion (.33 cup)

- Red bell peppers (.5 cup)

- Garlic (1 tbsp.)

- Dry white wine (2 tbsp.)

- Canned tomatoes (1.5 cups)

- Lemon juice (2 tbsp.)

- Chicken broth (.25 cup)

- Tabasco sauce (.25 tsp.)

- Black pepper and salt (.25 each or to your liking)

- Heavy cream (.25 cup)

- Thinly sliced scallions (.25 cup)

The Grits:

- Milk (1 cup)

- Grits (.5 cup)

- Water (1 cup)

- Pepper and salt (to your liking)

- Butter (1 tbsp.)

Preparation Technique:

1. Dab the shrimp dry using a paper towel and dust them using the Old Bay. Set it aside for now.

2. Select the sauté function and prepare the bacon for three minutes and set it aside to drain.

3. Mince and sauté the peppers, garlic, and onions in the bacon fat for about two to three minutes.

4. Pour in the wine to deglaze the pan and remove the tasty bits, simmering until most of the wine is evaporated.

5. Pour in lemon juice, tomatoes, pepper, salt, and hot sauce.

6. Place the trivet into the Instant Pot. Add the mixture into a medium container to fit inside the pot.

7. Whisk the milk, cornmeal, water, pepper, and salt. Place the bowl in the cooker and securely close the lid. Set the timer on manual function for ten minutes.

8. Natural-release the steam (10-15 min.), and open the Instant Pot.

9. Remove the cornmeal dish and trivet.

10. Mix in the shrimp and close the lid for the shrimp to heat in the keep-warm mode.

11. Butter the cornmeal and toss it.

12. After the shrimp has warmed ten minutes, open the lid and switch to the sauté function and add the cream.

13. Toss in bacon and scallions to reheat and serve with the prepared cornmeal, yummy.

Shrimp Scampi

Serving Yields: 15

Points Allotted - Smart Points: 11

Prep & Cooking Time: 15 minutes

Nutritional Macros Per Serving:

- **Calories**: 432
- **Protein Count**: 27 g
- **Fat Content**: 16 g
- **Carbs**: 13.5 g

List of Ingredients Needed:

- Shrimp (2 lb.)
- Olive oil (2 tbsp.)
- Pastured butter/Kerry gold (2 tbsp.)
- Homemade chicken stock (.5 cup)
- White wine (.5 cup)
- Gluten-free pasta (1 lb.)
- Fresh lemon juice (1 tbsp.)
- Black pepper & sea salt
- Optional for Garnish: Parsley

Preparation Technique:

1. Heat the Instant Pot using the sauté mode. Add the oil. Mince and add in the garlic to sauté until it's fragrant. Pour in the chicken stock and wine to deglaze the browned bits.

2. Add in the shrimp and set the Instant Pot to meat/stew for one minute.

3. Natural-release the pressure five minutes and quick-release the rest of the pressure.

4. Mix the fixings and serve with a spritz of lemon, pepper, and salt.

Shrimp With Beans & Rice

Serving Yields: 4

Points Allotted - Smart Points: 1

Prep & Cooking Time: 35 minutes

Nutritional Macros Per Serving:

- **Calories**: 276

- **Protein Count**: 32.5 g

- **Fat Content**: 11.5 g

- **Carbs**: 31 g

List of Ingredients Needed:

- Low-sodium vegetable broth (1.5 cups)

- Rice (1 cup)

- Minced garlic (2 tbsp.)

- Butter (.25 cup)

- Cooked shrimp (1 lb.)

- Black beans (1 can)

- Dried cilantro (to taste)

Preparation Technique:

1. Rinse and drain the beans.

2. Select the sauté mode and add the butter and rice to the Instant Pot.

3. Sauté for two to three minutes until lightly browned. Shake in the salt, pepper, and garlic, stirring for another two minutes.

4. Stir in the beans, broth, and shrimp.

5. Seal the valve and close the lid. Adjust the time for four to five minutes. Natural-release the pressure for eight to ten minutes after the buzzer goes off.

6. Open the top and add the shrimp on a platter and sprinkle with cilantro before serving.

10-Minute Instant Pot Salmon

Serving Yields: 4

Points Allotted - Smart Points: 6

Prep & Cooking Time: 25 minutes

Nutritional Macros Per Serving:

- **Calories**: 257
- **Protein Count**: 14 g
- **Fat Content**: 19 g
- **Carbs**: 6 g

List of Ingredients Needed:

- Medium lemon (3)
- Water (.75 cup)
- Salmon fillet (4)
- Fresh dill weed (1 bunch)
- Unsalted butter (1 tbsp.)
- Ground black pepper and salt (.25 tsp. each)
- Raw brown rice (1 cup)
- Green beans (4 cups)

Preparation Technique:

1. Drizzle the Instant Pot with about ¼ of the juice squeezed from the lemon and ¾ cup of water.

2. Add the fillets onto the steamer basket. Drizzle them with more lemon and more dill.

3. Securely close the lid and set the timer for five minutes.

4. When it buzzes, quick-release the steam pressure and serve with a bit of butter, fresh dill, salt, and pepper.

Wine-Marinated Shrimp

Serving Yields: 3

Points Allotted - Smart Points: 5

Prep & Cooking Time: 17 minutes

Nutritional Macros Per Serving:

- **Calories**: 153
- **Protein Count**: 16 g
- **Fat Content**: 6.5 g
- **Carbs**: 8 g

List of Ingredients Needed:

- Lemon juice (1 tbsp.)
- Lemon zest (.5 tsp.)
- Cilantro (2 tbsp.)
- Salt (.5 tbsp.)
- Ground ginger (.5 tsp.)
- Olive oil (1 tbsp.)
- White wine (.25 cup)
- Apple cider vinegar (2 tbsp.)
- Brown sugar (1 tsp.)
- Garlic (.5 tbsp.)
- Nutmeg (1 tsp.)
- Water (1 cup)
- Shrimp (5.5 lb.)
- Parsley (1 cup)

Preparation Technique:

1. Peel and devein the shrimp. Chop the parsley and cilantro.

2. Mix the vinegar, juice, garlic, lemon zest, white wine, salt, and sugar in a mixing container. Stir until the salt and sugar have dissolved.

3. Mix in the shrimp and add the cilantro and parsley. Stir and add the oil, ginger, water, and nutmeg. Marinate for about 15 minutes.

4. Add the shrimp mixture into the Instant Pot and close the lid.

5. Set the timer (manual) for eight minutes. When the timer buzzes, quick release the pressure and op the lid to serve.

Desserts

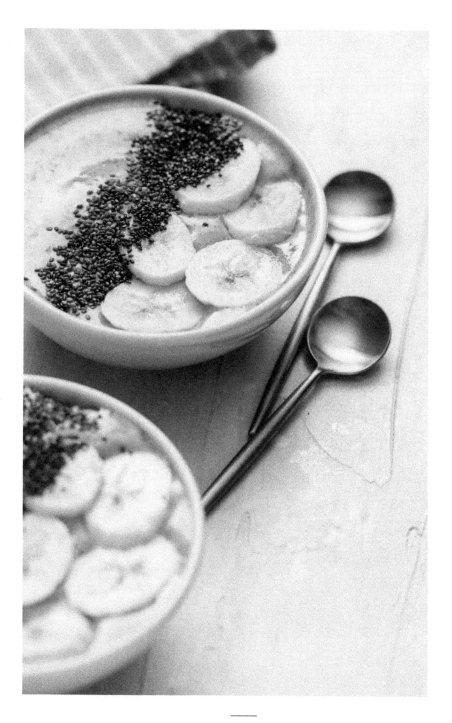

Applesauce

Serving Yields: 8

Points Allotted - Smart Points: 0

Prep & Cooking Time: 40 minutes

Nutritional Macros Per Serving:

- **Calories**: 88

- **Protein Count**: - g

- **Fat Content**: - g

- **Carbs**: 23 g

List of Ingredients Needed:

- Apples (3 lb.)

- Water (4 tbsp.)

- Cinnamon (.5-1 tsp.)

- Salt (1 pinch)

- Optional: Sweetener of choice

Preparation Technique:

1. Leave the peel on or off, but remove the cores and chop/slice into chunks.

2. Toss the apples, cinnamon, and water into the Instant Pot.

3. Securely close the top and set the timer for five minutes using high pressure.

4. When the timer beeps, natural-release the pressure (10-15 min.).

5. Open the Instant Pot and add the sweetener and pinch of salt.

6. Cream it using an immersion hand blender if you like a smooth textured applesauce.

Banana Cupcakes

Serving Yields: 6

Points Allotted - Smart Points: 8 /With frosting: 9

Prep & Cooking Time: 40 minutes

Nutritional Macros Per Serving:

- **Calories**: 314
- **Protein Count**: 6 g
- **Fat Content**: 9 g
- **Carbs**: 51 g

List of Ingredients Needed:

- Rice flour (1 cup)
- Ripe banana (1 mashed)
- Baking powder (1 tsp.)
- Baking soda (.25 tsp.)
- Salt (.25 tsp.)
- Egg (1)
- Vanilla (1 tsp.)
- Optional: Walnuts (.25 cup)
- Maple syrup (.5 cup)
- Almond milk (.25 cup)

Frosting Ingredients:

- Peanut butter (.25 cup)
- Cocoa powder (.25 tsp.)
- Maple syrup (2 tbsp.)

Preparation Technique:

1. Combine the cupcake fixings in a mixing bowl.

2. Dump the batter into silicone cupcake liners, filling the liners ¾ of the way full. You can also use ramekins or small glass jars to make mini cakes. Cover the container with foil.

3. Add 1.5 cups water to the bottom of the Instant Pot. Insert the trivet or a silicone steaming basket.

4. Carefully place the cupcakes on the trivet.

5. Close the lid and turn the pressure valve to sealing. Cook on high pressure for 25 minutes. Natural-release when it's done.

6. Remove the cupcakes and let them cool. If any condensation built-up on the cakes, dab them using a towel to dab it off.

7. While the cupcakes are cooling, mix the frosting. Spread or pipe the frosting onto the cakes before serving.

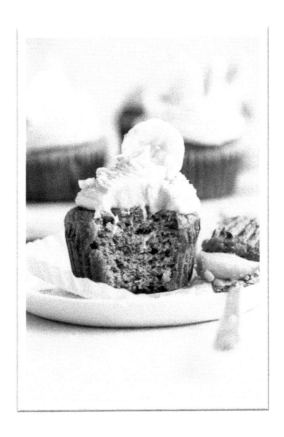

Chocolate Chip Cannolis

Serving Yields: 8

Points Allotted - Smart Points: 4

Prep & Cooking Time: 1 hour 15 minutes

Nutritional Macros Per Serving:

- **Calories**: 126

- **Protein Count**: 4 g

- **Fat Content**: 2 g

- **Carbs**: 12 g

List of Ingredients Needed:

- Reduced-fat ricotta cheese (1 cup + 2 tbsp.)

- Light whipped topping (half of 1 container)

- Powdered sugar (3 tbsp.)

- Almond extract (.75 tsp.)

- Fresh orange zest (.25 to .5 tsp.)

- Finely chopped dark chocolate (.75 oz.)

- Vanilla pizzelle cookies (8)

Preparation Technique:

1. Place the ricotta cheese into a cheesecloth in a strainer over a bowl to drain any excess liquids for an hour in the fridge.

2. Meanwhile, toss the rest of the fixings, omitting the cookies, in a mixing bowl and blend.

3. Dump the mixture into a bag with the tip cut to allow you to pipe it into your cannolis.

4. Microwave each pizzelle cookie individually for about 20 seconds.

5. You will want to form your cannoli with your fingers as soon as you remove it from the microwave. Let it cool. They will hold their new form.

6. Fill the cookies with the filling and sprinkle with the chocolate.

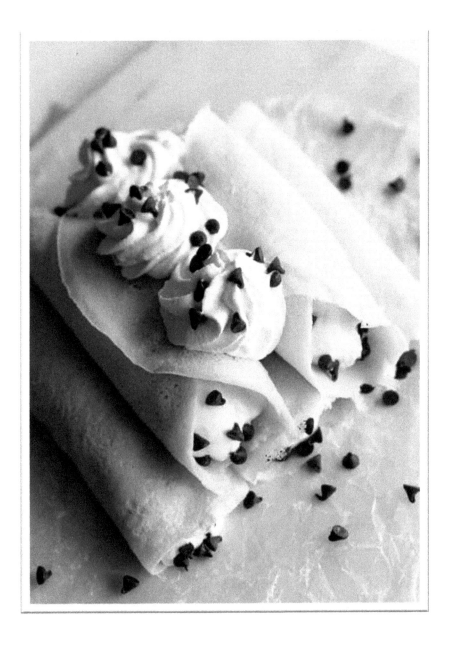

Delicious Apple Cake

Serving Yields: 8

Points Allotted - Smart Points: 6

Prep & Cooking Time: 40 minutes

Nutritional Macros Per Serving:

- **Calories**: 140

- **Protein Count**: 4 g

- **Fat Content**: 2 g

- **Carbs**: 10 g

List of Ingredients Needed:

- All-purpose flour (2 cups)

- Oats (1 cup)

- Sugar substitute suitable for baking (.5 cup)

- Salt (.25 tsp.)

- Baking soda (.25 tsp.)

- Cinnamon (2 tsp.)

- Vanilla extract (1 tsp.)

- Unsweetened applesauce (.5 cup)

- Diced apples - ex. Honeycrisp (2 cups)

- Unsweetened almond milk - original or vanilla (.5 cup)

Preparation Technique:

1. Place the trivet and one cup of water into the Instant Pot liner.

2. Spray a bowl that fits into the Instant Pot with a cooking oil spray.

3. Combine all of the fixings in a large mixing bowl and stir until well combined.

4. Pour it into the prepared bowl and place it onto the trivet in the Instant Pot liner.

5. Securely close the lid.

6. Set it to the Cake function for 25 minutes. When it's complete, natural-release the pressure for 5 minutes.

7. Release the remaining pressure, remove and serve.

Healthy Lava Cake

Serving Yields: 4

Points Allotted - Smart Points: 13

Prep & Cooking Time: 15 minutes

Nutritional Macros Per Serving:

- **Calories**: 298

- **Protein Count**: 5 g

- **Fat Content**: 16 g

- **Carbs**: 22 g

List of Ingredients Needed:

- Eggs (2)

- Ghee or butter (4 tbsp.)

- Dark chocolate pieces (.25 cup)

- Coconut milk (4 tbsp.)

- Rice flour (.33 cup)

- Salt (.25 tsp.)

- Honey (1 tbsp.)

- Baking powder (.5 tsp.)

- Cocoa powder (1 tbsp.)

- Optional: Additional dark chocolate for the center

Preparation Technique:

1. Add the dark chocolate and ghee in a microwave-safe dish. Melt it in the microwave using 30-second increments until its melted (no more than one minute).

2. Whisk in the remaining fixings into the melted chocolate and butter.

3. Lightly grease four ramekins with coconut oil.

4. Fill each of the ramekins ¾ of the way with batter. Cover each ramekin with foil.

5. Add the trivet/ or a steamer basket to the bottom of the Instant Pot with 1.5 cups of water. Arrange the ramekins on top of the trivet with three on the bottom and one stacked on top in the center.

6. Lock the top into place and turn the pressure valve to sealing. Cook the lava cakes on high pressure for four to five minutes (4 minutes will leave the center very gooey, while 5 minutes will have a little more cake texture around the center).

7. Release the pressure using the quick-release method.

8. Serve while hot. Top with coconut whipped cream or fresh banana ice cream.

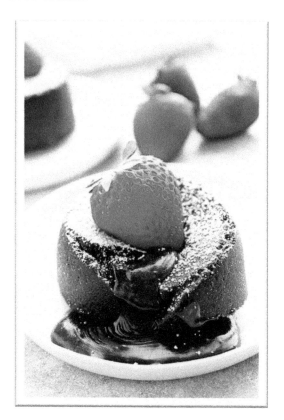

IP Cheesecake

Serving Yields: 6

Points Allotted - Smart Points: 4

Prep & Cooking Time: 55 minutes

Nutritional Macros Per Serving:

- **Calories**: 173

- **Protein Count**: 14 g

- **Fat Content**: 5 g

- **Carbs**: 19 g

List of Ingredients Needed:

The Filling:

- Cottage cheese (2 cups)

- Greek yogurt plain or vanilla (.5 cup)

- Eggs (2)

- Honey (3 tbsp.)

- Rice flour (1 tbsp.)

- Vanilla extract (1 tsp.)

- Strawberries sliced (.5 cup)

The Crust:

- Oatmeal (.5 cup)

- Honey (1 tbsp.)

- Butter - melted (1 tbsp.)

Preparation Technique:

1. In a food processor or blender, mix the crust fixings for two to three minutes until the oats are chopped

2. Pour the crust mixture into the bottom of a six-inch springform pan lined with wax paper. Press firmly to form a crust on the bottom.

3. Wash out the blender and fill it with the filling ingredients.

4. Blend the filling for five minutes until it is smooth. The mixture will be a little watery.

5. Pour the filling into the springform pan. Tightly cover the pan with foil to prevent water from getting the pan.

6. Pour two cups water in the bottom of the Instant Pot and add the trivet on the bottom with the handle up. Carefully insert the cheesecake into the Instant Pot.

7. Set the cooker using the manual function to cook on high pressure for 35 minutes. Let the pressure release naturally. Remove the cheesecake and let it rest in the refrigerator overnight.

8. When ready to serve top with fresh sliced strawberries.

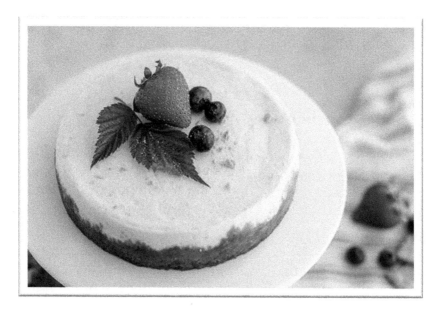

Key Lime Custard Bites

Serving Yields: 7

Points Allotted - Smart Points: 5

Prep & Cooking Time: 40 minutes

Nutritional Macros Per Serving:

- **Calories**: 300

- **Protein Count**: 6 g

- **Fat Content**: 20 g

- **Carbs**: 28 g

List of Ingredients Needed:

- Unsweetened almond milk (1 cup)

- Honey (.5 cup)

- Unflavored gelatin (1 tbsp.)

- Arrowroot powder or cornstarch (4 tbsp.)

- Key lime juice (.5 cup- about 10 key limes)

- Egg yolks (3)

The Crust:

- Peanuts (.5 cup)

- Coconut oil (.5 tbsp.)

Optional Coconut Whipped Cream:

- Coconut milk - refrigerated - so it's cold (1 can)

- Optional: Stevia (1 tsp.)

Preparation Technique:

1. In a food processor/hand mixer, mix all the ingredients for the filling.

2. Grease the silicone egg bite mold cups. Pour the filling into each cup ¾ of the way full. Tightly cover the silicone mold with foil.

3. Add 1.5 cups of water to the Instant Pot insert. Place the trivet at the bottom, and add the silicone mold onto the trivet.

4. Close the top and set the timer for 35 minutes using the high-pressure function.

5. Natural-release the built-up pressure. Remove the silicone mold from the Instant Pot.

6. Let the pies settle on the counter for one hour before adding the crust or moving to the fridge. They will be jiggly at this point.

7. In a food processor, crush the peanuts and coconut oil (20 seconds).

8. Spoon the peanut crust over each lime bite and gently pat it down. Cover the lime bites with foil and chill in the fridge overnight.

9. When you are ready to serve, pop out of the mold, place them on a place crust side down, and top with homemade coconut whipped cream and key lime slices.

Preparation Technique: *Coconut Whipped Cream:*

1. Open the can of cold coconut cream and separate the milk from the cream. (The cream is solid, and the milk is watery.)

2. Place the cream in a chilled bowl and add the stevia.

3. Beat the coconut cream with a hand mixer for one to two minutes until the coconut cream is soft and has a whipped cream texture.

4. Store in the fridge until you're ready to use it, but be sure to use it the same day you make it.

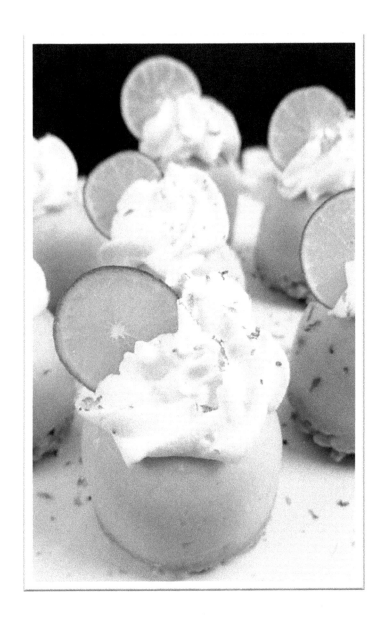

Pumpkin Fluff

Serving Yields: 8

Points Allotted - Smart Points:

Green: 4/Blue: 4/ Purple: 4

Prep & Cooking Time: 10 minutes

Nutritional Macros Per Serving:

- **Calories**: 155

- **Protein Count**: 2 g

- **Fat Content**: 2 g

- **Carbs**: 35 g

List of Ingredients Needed:

- Skim milk (1 cup)

- Sugar-free vanilla pudding mix (1 box)

- Canned pumpkin (15 oz.)

- Sugar-free Cool Whip (8 oz.)

- Pumpkin pie spice (1 tsp.)

- Cinnamon (1 tsp.)

Preparation Technique:

1. Add the pudding mix in a mixing bowl and pour in the milk. Beat the mixture for two minutes.

2. Stir in the pumpkin mix, and spices, omitting the Cool Whip.

3. When it is all well mixed, fold in the Cool Whip to serve.

Conclusion

I hope you have tried at least a few of the new recipes in your new copy of Weight Loss Instant Pot Freestyle Cookbook Recipes. Experiment with your favorites and show off your skills at the next family gathering or another special event! Before closing, let's just see how many healthy choices you will make by cooking with the Instant Pot.

Use the Instant Pot to prepare your meals in advance. The machine automatically activates the keep warm function after each cooking cycle. This allows you to prepare meals in the morning so that you can come home to a warm dinner. Or, set up the Instant Pot before going to bed so that breakfast is cooked when you wake up.

Preserve the Nutrients

You can use your pressure-cooking techniques using the Instant Pot to ensure the heat is evenly and quickly distributed. It is not essential to immerse the food into the water. You will provide plenty of water in the cooker for efficient steaming. You will also be saving the essential vitamins and minerals. The food won't become oxidized by the exposure of air or heat. Enjoy those fresh green veggies with their natural and vibrant colors.

The cooking elements help keep the foods fully sealed, so the steam and aromas don't linger throughout your entire home. That is a plus, especially for items such as cabbage, which throws out a distinctive aroma.

You will find that beans and whole grains will have a softer texture and will have an improved taste. The meal will be cooked consistently since the Instant Pot provides even heat distribution.

Programming Benefits

You have the operational buttons that perform different tasks to save you time in the kitchen. You can choose from the preset programs or follow guidelines as provided in your particular recipe. Each function will refine your search to prepare a variety of foods from rare to well done, depending on your personal preferences.

Save Time & Energy

You will be using much less water, and the pot is fully insulated, making it more energy-efficient when compared to boiling or steaming your foods on the stovetop. It is also less expensive than using a microwave, not to mention how much more flavorful the food will be when prepared in the Instant Pot cooker.

You can delay the cooking of your food items so you can plan ahead of time. You won't need to stand around as you await your meal. You can reduce the cooking time by reducing the 'hands-on' time. Just leave for work or a day of activities, and you will come home to a special treat.

Difference Between Pressure Cooking vs. Other Cooking Methods

Pressure cooking means that you can (on average) cook meals 75% faster than boiling/braising on the stovetop or baking/roasting in a conventional oven.

This is especially helpful for vegan meals that entail the use of dried beans, legumes, and pulses. Instead of pre-soaking these ingredients for hours before use, you can pour them directly into the Instant Pot, add water, and pressure cook these for several minutes. However, always follow your recipe carefully since they have been tested for accuracy.

Finally, if you found this book useful in any way, a review on Amazon is always appreciated!